Nursing M and Their Psychiatric Mental Health Applications

Joyce J. Fitzpatrick, PhD, FAAN, RN
Ann L. Whall, PhD, FAAN, RN
Ruth L. Johnston, PhD, RN
Judith A. Floyd, MS, RN

343879

Robert J. Brady Co., Bowie, Maryland 20715
A Prentice-Hall Publishing and Communications Company

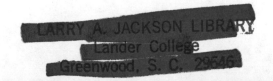

Executive Producer: Richard Weimer
Production Editor: Paula Aldrich
Art Director: Don Sellers, A.M.I.

Nursing Models and Their Psychiatric Mental Health Applications.

Library of Congress Cataloging in Publication Data

Nursing models and their psychiatric mental health applications.

Includes bibliographies and index.
Contents: Relevance of psychiatric mental
health nursing theories to nursing models /
Ruth L. Johnston and Joyce J. Fitzpatrick—
The crisis perspective / Joyce J. Fitzpatrick—
Individual psychotherapy / Ruth J. Johnston—
[etc.]
1. Psychiatric nursing—Addresses, essays,
lectures. I. Fitzpatrick, Joyce J.
[DNLM: 1. Psychiatric nursing. 2. Models,
Psychological. WY 160 N9765]
RC440.N88   610.73'68   81-10108
ISBN 0-89303-026-0   AACR2

Prentice-Hall International, Inc., London
Prentice-Hall of Australia, Pty., Ltd., Sydney
Prentice-Hall of India Private Limited, New Delhi
Prentice-Hall of Japan, Inc., Tokyo
Prentice-Hall of Southeast Asia Pte. Ltd., Singapore
Whitehall Books, Limited, Petone, New Zealand

Printed in the United States of America

82 83 84 85 86 87 88 89 90 91 92   10 9 8 7 6 5 4 3 2 1

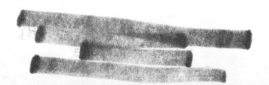

CONTENTS

PREFACE

At the onset of a task, it is probably just as important to identify what one is *not* attempting to accomplish, as what one *is* attempting to do. With this in mind, we began with a clear understanding of what this text would not be. We believe that there are many comprehensive psychiatric mental health nursing texts available today, providing adequate coverage of general information. What we believe is not adequately addressed, not only by the texts, but by psychiatric mental health nursing in general, is the use of nursing models to assess, evaluate, and reformulate existing borrowed theories.

We believe that the nursing models, in general, (such as those of King, Orem, Rogers, and Roy) describe prevailing views for the discipline of nursing with regard to person, environment, health, and nursing. These nursing models are currently developed to a level where concepts are at times defined operationally but the relationships between concepts have not been explicitly developed. Consequently, there is potential for development of these models into various levels of theory, with guidelines for practice yet to be developed. What is available to guide the practice of psychiatric mental health nursing has, for the most part, been "borrowed" from other disciplines. These borrowed theories, although applied in individual ways by individual nurses, have not led to a distinct psychiatric mental health nursing approach, i.e., distinct from other therapeutic disciplines also utilizing the same theories. Identity problems abound as psychiatric mental health nurses have asked of themselves over time, "How are we distinct or different? Is there a difference?"

We believe the difference is there, but that it has not been well explicated. What is needed now is a merger of prevailing nursing views, a merger of the nursing models with existing psychiatric mental health theories. We believe the nursing models should be used to reformulate or change the existing theories for the purposes of nursing.

What of the ethics and methods involved in reformulation of borrowed theory? We agree with those philosophers of science, such as Abraham Kaplan, who posit that concepts and theories are not "owned" by any one discipline, but rather, that each discipline has a right and a responsibility to select from the available knowledge, and to modify and reformulate those theoretical positions to its own purposes. In this initial effort of reformulation, selected concepts of existing theories, as well as some of the more essential propositions, are reformed according to a nursing model. Others may continue this work, thus leading to a fuller reformulation of the borrowed theories. However, full reformulation of the borrowed theories is not possible until congruencies and incongruencies with the nursing models are identified.

Throughout this work, we present a variety of nursing models but are selective in the reformulation of existing theories. Further, there is no attempt to include *all* the therapeutic modalities with which psychiatric mental health nursing is concerned. In this initial effort, only approaches to individuals and families are considered. In the last chapter we present a less well known theoretical perspective. We have done this to demonstrate the efficacy of this approach, not only with well developed theories, but also for use with less well developed theoretical positions. We believe that the future of nursing science has never been brighter. As nursing continues to develop its own approaches to person, environment, and health, a distinct theoretical base of nursing practice becomes more and more evident.

Each chapter maintains a similar format in that the major concepts and propositions of the existing theory are identified. The way in which the concepts of nursing, person, health, and environment, identified within the nursing model, as well as within the existing theory, are then addressed. Finally, ways in which the existing theory might be reformulated according to the nursing model are developed. Practice examples further explain the reformulations. We hope that these beginning attempts to undertake the necessary reformulations will stimulate similar attempts by psychiatric mental health nursing practitioners.

Ann L. Whall

FOREWORD

In this work the authors present an array of theoretical perspectives, drawn from the nursing and non-nursing literature, for application in nursing practice. Contemporary nursing models are summarized, similarities and differences among them are set forth, and relationships to nursing research, education, and practice are indicated. The profession of nursing is broadening the base of scientific knowledge that nurses use in their practice. This work contributes significantly to that effort by providing a broad range of conceptual frameworks and suggesting their relevance in the practices of nurses.

The profession of nursing is gradually moving away from the "medical model" toward conceptual models that are more relevant to nursing practice. This transition is consonant with an enlarging interest in nursing research, increasing effort in understanding phenomena of direct concern in nursing practice, greater sophistication of nurses in theory application in nursing practice, and other trends which mark the growing professionalization of nursing. The development of nursing models, and other conceptual frameworks for practice, as described in this work, are aspects of the intellectual ferment taking place during this transition from medically-oriented nursing care toward nurse-directed nursing practice.

In the past three decades the role of nurse has expanded and become more definitive. Previously, the knowledge base used by nurses, drawn from basic and applied sciences, consisted primarily in intrapersonal theories. Physical care and within-person phenomena were the major focus of nursing practice. Today, the focus of nursing, as set forth in nurse practice acts, requires a broader base of scientific knowledge for the effective practice of nursing. Interpersonal and systems theories, crisis theory, and rhythm theory, as presented by the authors in this work, are necessary for nurses practicing in expanded roles. Two modalities of treatment now common in the practice of nursing—psychotherapy and family therapy—which are also described in this work, are instances of the expanded role that nurses are taking.

While the emphasis in this book is on the application of contemporary theory to psychiatric mental health nursing, this text has wider significance. Problems in living are seen not only in the mentally ill but, in some degree, in all persons who seek the help that nurses provide.

Hildegard E. Peplau, RN, EdD, FAAN

1 RELEVANCE OF PSYCHIATRIC MENTAL HEALTH NURSING THEORIES TO NURSING MODELS

Ruth L. Johnston and Joyce J. Fitzpatrick

For many years, psychiatric mental health nursing practice has been dominated by the medical model. Practitioners were taught and supervised mainly by physicians. At the same time, throughout the history of nursing, leaders have emerged to provide impetus to the development of psychiatric mental health nursing based on nursing as an independent discipline. This nursing perspective is concerned with broad health aspects of the human condition and the experience of life.

Notable in the transition from physician-directed psychiatric mental health nursing practice toward the emergence of theory-based practice were Theresa G. Muller and Hildegard Peplau. They made significant contributions in advancing the role of the nurse as a primary psychiatric mental health therapist.

Muller was influential in obtaining recognition of nursing as the fourth professional discipline in mental health. Federal assistance was therefore available for the establishment of graduate programs in nursing within universities.[1] Muller established four of the early programs leading to masters degrees in psychiatric nursing and was Director of Graduate Studies for the first such program at Catholic University. She subsequently established and directed programs at Boston University, Indiana University, and the University of Nebraska. Her emphasis was on the need for graduate education, and on interdisciplinary preparation as a means of establishing collaborative interdisciplinary practice. Clinical practice, rather than functional specialization, was a clear emphasis in these programs (Muller 1950).

Although perhaps most significantly influenced by Jungian analytical psychology, Muller was a strong proponent of the need to explore alternative theories in the development of professional practice. Her teaching reflected the recognition of the contributions of Freud, Rank,

---

[1] The National Mental Health Act of 1946, enacted in response to the overwhelming numbers of psychiatric casualties encountered both in selection of men for service, and in response to combat, provided funds for graduate education in nursing, psychiatry, psychology and social work.

and Adler, as well as the newer emphasis on group approaches, e.g., group dynamics, group therapy, and psychodrama (Muller 1950).

Peplau made a major contribution to the profession of nursing and the move toward theory-based practice through her book, *Interpersonal Relations in Nursing* (Peplau 1952). Her impact on graduate education in psychiatric nursing at Teachers College, Columbia University, and for many years at Rutgers, the State University of New Jersey, is well known. Sills noted that a major contribution of Peplau was the methodologically disciplined nature of the educational experience. Through Peplau's mentorship, students were "diverse yet similar, wedded to a practice/theory experiential model of clinical work . . ." (Sills 1978, p. 124). The extent of the Peplau impact on research and publications in the decades since the publication of her 1952 book is documented by Sills (1977).

Additional benchmarks in the transition to theory-based practice can be seen in the work of Gwen Tudor in "Sociopsychiatric nursing approach to intervention in a problem of mutual withdrawal on a mental hospital ward" (Tudor 1952). This was the first research publication in psychiatric nursing. It is noteworthy for its reflection of the transition from the within-person focus to an interpersonal approach (Sills 1978).

Theoretical formulations such as the psychoanalytic perspective of nursing have been developed from broad perspectives of man, health, and/or environment. These formulations have been specific in their descriptions of mental health and illness. This heritage of breadth in theory, resulting from identification with disciplines other than nursing, has limited the unification of theoretical orientations in psychiatric mental health nursing. There is a current need for emphasis on theory-based practice within the mainstream of the discipline of nursing. The focus of this text is on the analysis of selected broad-based theoretical formulations that have guided psychiatric mental health nursing practice. These existing theories are reformulated in the light of certain nursing conceptual models. Particular attention is given to the conceptual models developed by King, Orem, Roy, and Rogers.

RELATIONSHIP OF CONCEPTUAL FRAMEWORKS TO THEORY DEVELOPMENT

Nye and Berardo (1966) define theory as characterized by systematically organized, law-like propositions in adequate number relating to a given problem to permit the formulation of significant hypotheses with a high rate of positive affirmation. Using this specific definition as the criterion, they were unable to describe one theory in the area of family in which the propositions are law-like. Similar criticisms have been offered of the nursing "theories" or conceptual frameworks such as those included here.

Conceptual frameworks may be considered a first step in theory building, introducing an element of orderliness into the research process and findings. Further, conceptual frameworks can facilitate the research process by providing a range of ideas for hypotheses generation. A review of a conceptual framework should suggest variables that otherwise might be overlooked. Conceptual frameworks can be understood as necessary and significant to the theory building and research processes.

The traditional approach to research, that of individual researchers undertaking studies in isolation, often without clearly stated conceptualizations and measures that are comparable with those used in other studies, has limited the effectiveness of both research and theory building. This same approach has been predominant in professional nursing practice. This has restricted the development of unified theoretical approaches to guide practice.

Conceptual frameworks differ from theories more in their underlying assumptions than in their concepts. Conceptual frameworks are often useful for data classification and for theory development. Such conceptual schemes can integrate disparate research findings from which hypotheses can be derived. Aldous (1970) identifies a need for replication and use of existing conceptual frameworks, not to preclude the addition of novel concepts and hypotheses, but to continue to focus on those issues from which the crucial variables have not yet been discovered.

Components of Conceptual Frameworks

Accepting conceptual frameworks as the recommended strategy for theory development, further assistance in developing understanding of the components of the conceptual framework is facilitated by attention to five categories of concepts presented by Nye and Berardo (1966):

1. Type of behavior treated
2. Social space in which it occurs
3. Time dimensions with which it deals
4. Substantive foci of research
5. Basic assumptions which underlie research and action

In nursing, the existing conceptual frameworks have not been used to view extant theories in terms of the conceptual relationships. For example, Whall (1980) noted that nursing's approach to families is characterized by the tendency of nursing practitioners and researchers to accept family theories "as is." She also expressed a concern regarding the need to evaluate these existing theories in terms of the syntax of the discipline of nursing, and accept, modify, or reject on the basis of appropriateness to nursing. Within the scope of that admonition, she reiterated the central concepts that are dealt with by all nursing models; person, environment, health, and nursing (Whall 1980). The underlying assumptions for dealing with these concepts will be explored.

Hill and Mattessich (1979) presented issues in which they compare two dominant paradigms, and a third emerging one. The paradigms are mechanistic and organismic, and the third, variously called relational, transactional, dialectical, and dynamic interactional, represents attempts to reach beyond the irreconcilable nature of the first two to relate them. Several of these issues will be described, and then used as a base for further exploring the nursing conceptual frameworks. Positions on these issues correlate with positions on openness of systems, and on organismic versus mechanistic views of the nature of man. This difference in open and closed systems models is elaborated also by Hultsch and Plemens (1979).

1. *External* versus *internal* locus of developmental change. Man as an actor involves the internal locus; man as a reactor involves the predominance of external stimulus for change.

2. *Reductionism* versus *emergence*. The mechanistic model is based upon an assumption of reductionism, assuming that any behavioral skill can be reduced to a simpler, more elementary form. On the other hand, characteristic of the organismic model is the concept of emergence. In the concept of emergence, later forms cannot be reduced to earlier forms. The symbolic level of hierarchical order makes reductionism incompatible with systems theory.

3. *Universality* versus *relativity*. The organismic view embraces the universality of development; that individuals evolve through an invariant sequence of developmental stages common to all human beings. The dialectic model is compatible with the biologic universality, but accepts also the concepts of culturally variant and genetic-experiential uniqueness. The mechanistic position, the reactive model, would likely assume that development proceeds uniquely for each individual. Relativity in development would be manifest in a description of individuals as culture-bound.

4. *Unidirectionality* versus *bidirectionality*. As would be anticipated with a conceptualization of emergent rather than reductionistic, unidirectionality is characteristic of the organismic model.

Since all of the major nursing conceptual frameworks (i.e., King 1971, Orem 1971, Rogers 1970, 1980, Roy 1971) declare an underlying assumption encompassing systems theory, exploration of the assumptions involved is an appropriate step in the exploration and reformulation of other theories borrowed by nursing.

SYSTEMS THEORY:

A REVIEW   Although the concept of systems dates back to the fifteenth century, the development of systems theory is largely credited to von Bertalanffy. He defines a system as "a set of units with relationships among them" (von Bertalanffy 1969, p. 68). The need for a systems approach was expressed as the increasing complexity rendering the causal model inadequate to explain or predict the responses of living organisms. This was further elaborated by Miller (1969), who speaks of living systems as being made of matter and energy organized by information.

Systems literature provides evidence of the emergence of systems theory from the "closed systems" concepts to "open systems" concepts with overlapping and confusing definitions resulting as attempts are made to explain increasingly complex phenomena. The concept of hierarchical order best seems to describe the systems theorist's idea of the universe, the totality of experience. The major levels in the hierarchy are the inorganic, living, and symbolic worlds. Symbolic is the term to convey those activities, products, and interrelationships that form the superstructure of human culture and history. Those who accept this approach indicate that it is the symbolic level that makes it impossible to reduce human behavior to the animal level.

Characteristics of closed systems include:

1. A constant action-reaction between associated things;
2. A compensating factor which is provided by the system when the balance is upset;
3. An equal reaction for every action;
4. A tendency to remain in homeostasis once a system is established.

In a further attempt to understand the living organism as a system, cybernetics emerged, a science that specifically considers the application of control principles to the biological organism. Cybernetics proposes that randomly distributed objects or particles in a state of rhythmic oscillation can affect one another through interactions—a feedback of information that tends to stabilize the system. Two types of feedback can occur: negative feedback, which corrects the overdeviation in an error activated system; and positive feedback, deviation amplifying that can lead to breakdown of the system. Further elaboration of the concept of feedback led to negative feedback as morphostasis, positive feedback as morphogenosis. These same concepts are discussed by Maruyama (1963) as deviation counteracting (negative feedback) and deviation amplifying (positive feedback), both of which fall under the subject matter of cybernetics. Both are mutual-causal processes, but deviation counteracting processes are those that maintain homeostasis, and deviation amplifying are those in which deviation from homeostasis occurs as the second cybernetics. Rather than pressure to restore to equilibrium (negative feedback loop), positive reinforcement occurs which accelerates the deviation through a mutual causal process (Maruyama 1963).

This process offers an alternative to the usual causal model. Through this process, the law of causality is now revised to state that similar conditions may result in dissimilar products. This revision is made without the introduction of indeterminism and probabilism. When deviation amplifying mutual causal process is combined with indeterminism, a revision is necessary. The revision includes a small initial deviation, which is within the range of high probability, and may develop into a deviation of low probability—more specifically, a deviation that is very improbable within the framework of probabilistic un-idirectional causality (Maruyama 1963).

An additional classification of systems includes conceptual systems, developed by an investigator for purposes of study, and real systems (biological structures, solar systems). If perceived as closed systems, real systems do not exchange matter or energy. Intrusion thus increases the loss of organization and change in the direction of dissolution of the system. Closed systems are characterized by entropy (the running down of the system). Closed systems strive for homeostasis (for every action there is a reaction). If perceived as open systems, the response to intrusion is typically an elaboration or change in the structure to a higher, more complex level. Environmental interchange is an essential factor; open systems are characterized by negentropy, or increased complexity, diversity, and heterogeneity (Kaufman 1969).

In summary, the following assumptions underlie the systems view:

1. Normal differentiation in man implies progressive organization within an integrated whole or system;
2. The concept of hierarchical order seems to best describe the systems theorist's idea of the universe: inorganic, living, and symbolic;
3. The symbolic world includes culture and history and makes reductionistic approaches incompatible with systems theory.

ANALYSIS OF SELECTED
NURSING MODELS

The conceptual frameworks developed by King (1971), Orem (1971), Rogers (1970), and Roy (1976) are currently considered among those that provide models for the science of nursing. These models contain the basic elements of conceptual frameworks in the more abstract definition and have provided the organizational framework for derived theoretical models. The most frequently expressed objection to these conceptual models is that the posited relationships cannot be or have not been subjected to empirical test.

Despite the consistent and necessary focus on the differences identified in the theorists' conceptualizations, it is apparent that there are similar basic concepts incorporated in each of these models. Four such concepts have been identified: person, environment, health, and nursing (Fawcett 1978, 1980). It is proposed that these concepts, and the relationship that the nursing process is utilized in interaction with persons and their environments to assist them to achieve health, form the basis of the predominant perspective for the scientific discipline and the professional practice of nursing.

An attempt will be made to elucidate the similarities inherent in the conceptualizations. At the same time differences in conceptualizations will be noted. These similarities and differences will be explained in relation to the particular psychiatric mental health theories being studied for reformulation purposes. Rogers' conceptualization will be explored in more detail as this conceptual framework clearly reflects an open system perspective.

Each of these conceptual frameworks will be reviewed in terms of the five categories presented by Nye and Berardo (1966). Attention is also directed toward elucidation of the open or closed system assumptions included in each framework. Furthermore, the basic theoretical postulations are extracted from each of the conceptual frameworks. This presentation and initial analysis of the conceptual frameworks of King, Orem, Rogers, and Roy lay the foundation for the following chapters, i.e., the explication of relationships between the nursing models and selected psychiatric mental health theories.

Rogers' Unitary Man Model

Rogers' (1970) science of unitary man is based on conceptualizations of man-environment interaction characterized by rhythms throughout the developmental process, movement toward increasing complexity and diversity, and the changes in patterns and organization evidenced by changes in the associated wave patterns and rhythmic activity identifying the whole (Fitzpatrick 1980).

"Theory of synergistic man postulates phylogenetic and ontogentic developmental processes characterized by increasing complexity and diversity of pattern and organization. The process of human development is viewed as consistent with environmental changes, and variations in rhythmic patterns of man-environment interaction can be identified. Understanding of the developmental correlates of the evolutionary process is basic to a discussion of the emerging trends in human patterning" (Fitzpatrick, 1980 p. 148). These developmental correlates include: movement from a smaller human field through a larger one toward boundarylessness; movement from higher density through lower toward ethereal; movement from heaviness through lightness toward weightlessness; movement from pragmatic through imaginative toward visionary; movement from longer, lower frequency waves through shorter, higher frequency ones toward waves that seem continuous; movement from slower rhythms through faster rhythms toward rhythms that seem continuous; movement from slower motion through faster motion toward motionlessness; movement from a perception of time dragging through a perception of time racing toward timelessness; movement from sleeping through waking toward beyond waking states (altered states of consciousness); movement from less differentiation through more differentiation toward transcendence; movement from three-dimensional reality through four-dimensional reality toward multidimensional reality; and movement from shorter life spans through longer life spans toward transformation (Rogers 1970, 1980).

The science of synergistic man is defined as the study of the behavior of whole systems, behavior that cannot be predicted by behavior of the component functions taken separately. Behavioral manifestations of the life process are expressions of a unified whole having distinctive characteristics which cannot be dichotomized as mental or physical, as subjective or objective. The essential characteristic describing man as synergistic implies that the identity of man exists only in his wholeness.

Conceptualization of man as a field further describes his holistic nature. The human field is an open system characterized by pattern and organization, continuously interacting with the environment. Man and environment evolve as a totality, exchanging matter and energy in the dynamic evolutionary process. Man's life process is a becoming; evolving irreversibly and unidirectionally along the space-time continuum. The movement of the universal system, of man and environment, is goal directed and purposeful, continually evolving toward increasing complexity and diversity.

The human field and the environmental field can be described further by their pattern and organization, their structure and function, concepts and characteristics which refer to holistic behavior of open systems. Patterns reflecting various developmental stages can be identified. At the same time, the continuous repatterning of man and environment reflects the dynamic nature of the universe.

In summary, the assumptions on which the science of unitary man is based include:

1. Man is a unified whole possessing his own integrity and manifesting characteristics that are more than and different from the sum of his parts;
2. Man and environment are open systems, continually exchanging matter and energy with each other;

3. The life process evolves irreversibly and unidirectionally along the space time continuum;

4. Pattern and organization identify man and reflect his innovative wholeness;

5. Man is characterized by the capacity for abstraction and imagery, language and thought, sensation and emotion (Rogers 1970).

The principles of Rogers' model include focus on the inseparable man–environment open system as negentropic, innovative, and probabilistic.

> *Principle of Helicy:* The nature and direction of human and environmental change is continuously innovative, probabilistic, and characterized by increasing diversity of human field and environmental field pattern and organization emerging out of the continuous, mutual interaction between the fields and manifesting non-repeating rhythmicities.
>
> *Principle of Resonancy:* The human field and the environmental field are identified by wave pattern and organization manifesting continuous change from lower frequency, longer wave patterns to higher frequency, shorter wave patterns.
>
> *Principle of Complementarity:* Complementarity is characterized by a process of continuous mutual interaction between human and environmental fields (Rogers 1980).

The scientific principles derived from the conceptual model, i.e., helicy, resonancy, and complementarity (Rogers 1980), represent broad generalizations which are supported by experimental data, provide a foundation for the development of testable hypotheses. These principles describe the evolution of the life process as multidimensional, dynamic, and unidirectional. In addition, the life process in man is described as a symphony of rhythmical vibrations oscillating at various frequencies (Rogers 1970). In other words, the life process is an orderly, continuously changing, unending flow of wave patterns. This conceptualization has, as a unifying idea, rhythmic phenomena. Identified human and environmental rhythmic patterns include day and night rhythms, sleep-wake rhythms, emotional rhythms, changes in motion, and changes in perceptions of space time. This conceptualization of the rhythmic developmental progression is illustrated by the picket fence, with its identifiable, short, high-frequency rhythm of peaks and troughs. If viewed in rapid motion, the peaks and troughs, the waves and rhythms, are so fast that they seem continuous, suggesting a straight line or non-picket fence (Fitzpatrick 1980, p. 149).

From the perspective of the categories of concepts outlined by Nye and Berardo (1966), the Rogerian conceptual framework will be viewed from each category of concept outlined. First, in relation to the *type of behavior* treated, Rogers' principle of complementarity describes the continuous interaction process between human and environmental fields. Principles of helicy and resonancy describe more fully the nature of the man-environment interaction. Second, the *social space* within which it occurs is described as coextensive with the universe. Within this conceptual framework, man, a four-dimensional energy field, is embedded in environment, a four-dimensional energy field, coextensive with the universe. The open system is without boundaries, is probabilistic, and acausal. The *time dimension* with which this framework deals is described as nonlinear, unidirectional, and four dimensional. Four dimensionality is described as the transcendence of the time-space interaction. The *substantive focus* of this framework is the inseparable man-environment open system, negentropic, innovative, and probabilistic.

Viewing Rogers' conceptual framework from the paradigm of a development approach, it is apparent that this conceptual framework is incompatible with either psychoanalytic theory (mechanistic, reductionistic, reactive to inner locus of dynamic development, linear, causal, bidirectional) or behavior theory (mechanistic, reductionistic, reactive to outer locus of dynamic development, linear, causal, bidirectional). An open systems approach, such as that developed by Rogers, necessarily views the whole as more than, and different from, the sum of its parts, and as such, cannot be understood from the study of parts. The concepts of universality, unidirectionality, and emergence are compatible.

Perhaps the greatest congruence is apparent with the concepts characterizing the relatively new life span development family framework. Life span development refers to the increasing differentiation of personality structure and social competencies, recognition that increasing differentiation stimulates change in family organization, and that these changes in turn stimulate differentiation in development of child and adult personalities. Moves toward synthesis between organismic and mechanistic paradigms are evidenced. The dialectic model (or transactional) is compatible with all three views of humankind on the issue of universality versus relativity of development. It is biologically universal, culturally variant, and genetically-experientially unique. Hill et al. (1979) posit "high cross-cultural variability in the phenomenon of family development in the timing and duration of developmental processes, as well as in the age composition of family membership, but would hypothesize that ordering and sequence, and general shape of family development do approximate universality across cultures" (p. 187). Rogers' conceptualization differs from family development, and indeed, from family life span development, in the "openness" of the system. The family developmental conceptual framework tends to view the family system as semi-closed, with varying permeability of the boundaries, and in degree of linkages with external systems. Rogers' framework posits man-environment as a four-dimensional energy field, co-extensive with the universe. Boundaries exist only as arbitrarily defined for purposes of study.

The King Systems Model

King includes the basic concepts of person, perception, interpersonal relations, social systems, and health illness in her conceptual framework. Man is viewed as a total organism with continually evolving needs in the biologic, psychologic, and social realms. Man interacts with persons and things in his environment and functions within social systems. The individual's perception of the internal and external environment influences this interaction process. Health is defined as a dynamic state in the life cycle which implies adaptation to stresses in the internal and external environment through optimum use of one's resources to achieve maximum potential. Health includes aspects of the biophysical, the psychological, and the social elements. Nursing is a process of action, reaction, interaction, and transaction in which nurses assist individuals to meet their basic needs and to cope with health and illness (King 1968, 1971).

In summary, an analysis of the interrelationships posited in the theory yields the following propositional statements:

1. Man as a total (biopsychosocial) organism interacts with his internal and external environments.
2. Human behavior is understood in terms of personal, interpersonal, and social systems.
3. Man's personal system is characterized by perceptions of his environment that influence his interaction processes within the interpersonal and social systems.
4. Perceptions are temporally focused, i.e., man perceives and experiences based on his awareness of past and present and his predictions of the future; the flow of events in time follows an irreversible process which man understands to be time oriented.
5. Health is a dynamic state that implies continuous adaptation to stresses in the internal and external environment through use of one's resources.
6. Health is determined by man's functioning within the personal, interpersonal, and social realms at a given point in time.
7. Health includes internal and external aspects of the biophysical element, emotional and intelligence aspects of the psychological element, and the economic, ethnic, and religious aspects of the social element.
8. In health, physiological and psychological processes of the internal environment work in harmony to enable individuals to adjust to the continuous changes in the external environment.

9. Nursing is a process of interaction with individuals or groups to assist them in their present movement toward health through observations of the needs and behaviors related to personal (biopsychosocial), interpersonal (interpersonal relations, communication), and social (organization, status, role functioning) systems.

The King model is clearly incompatible with both the external *and* internal locus of developmental change. Neither is it compatible with the reductionistic or mechanistic approaches of psychoanalytic theory or behaviorism. The open system nature of this model necessitates an organismic, interactional, emergent approach. On the issue of universality versus relativity of development, the King model embraces both, characteristic of dialectic or transactional models in general. Unidirectionality rather than bidirectionality is implied in the temporal component, and the emergent nature of movement from action through interaction to transaction is the goal of the system. The degree of openness in this model is compatible with the communications theorists such as Watzlawick et al. (1967), who share an interactionist approach, but focus on families as the system unit.

First, in relation to *type of behavior treated*, King's personal, interpersonal, and social systems describe man's biopsychosocial nature in interaction with his internal and external environments. The perceptions that characterize his personal system influence his interaction process with the interpersonal and social systems. The *social space*, then, is the social system that defines the boundaries of the man-environment interaction. The *time dimension* is exemplified in man's perception of his experiences based on his awareness of the past and the present and his predictions of the future in the flow of events: an irreversible process which man understands to be time oriented. The *substantive focus* in this model is the relationship of the man-environment action, interaction, and transaction within the three systems.

The Orem Self Care Model

Concepts basic to Orem's conceptual model of nursing include holistic man and environment, health and self care. Basically, the individual is viewed as a composite unity functioning biologically, symbolically, and socially. The state of health is a reflection of the integrity of the whole, which may be described in relation to the component parts and the modes of functioning. Health is the capacity to live as a human being within one's physical, biologic, and social environments, achieving some measure of human life potential. Health must include that which makes man human (forms of mental life), operating in conjunction with physiologic mechanisms and a material structure (biologic life) and in relation to and interacting with other human beings (social life). According to Orem, the nursing focus is on the self care requirements of clients, i.e., when individuals need assistance with universal or health deviation self care activities, nursing intervention is appropriate (Orem 1971, Nursing Development Conference Group 1973).

The theoretical model can be summarized by the following derived propositional statements:

1. Man is a unity that can be viewed as functioning biologically, symbolically, and socially.
2. Man's functioning is linked to his environment and together they form an integrated functional system.
3. Health illness is a continuum which reflects man's interaction with his environment and is evidenced by behaviors related to cognition, biophysiological aspects, and social relationships.
4. Health related behaviors are directed toward man's need for self care whether universally required (universal self care) or required only in the event of illness, injury, or disease (health deviation self care).
5. Self care behaviors may be internal or external and are related to specific and combined properties of the human system in the biologic, symbolic, and social spheres of functioning.
6. Self care is the practice of activities that individuals personally initiate and perform on their own behalf in maintaining life, health, and well-being; the process of initiating self care includes decision making and deliberate action.
7. Variables that influence health and self care initiation include the health related state and powers of agency of the individual, i.e., mental development, personal maturity, social effectiveness, and competency in deliberate actions.
8. Activities of the self care agent are learned relative to the beliefs, habits, and practices that characterize the cultural way of life of the group to which the individual belongs and may include a wide range of alternative decisions and behaviors.
9. Self care actions are related to the nature and scope of changes in situations relevant to universal and health deviation self care, including demands imposed by changes in universal self care needs and demands imposed by the specific nature of health deviations.
10. Nursing agents intervene to provide therapeutic self care in supporting life processes, promoting normal functioning, maintaining normal growth, development, and maturation, and preventing or controlling disease processes.

The combination of a strong societal influence with the goal directed deliberative action of holistic man, within a system of interaction, makes either external or internal locus of developmental change, alone, incompatible with this theory. Organismic, rather than mechanistic orientation is implied, and the symbolic nature of man makes reductionism incompatible. There seems to be a strong emphasis on universality rather than relativity in the developmental process within this framework.

First, the *behavior* treated in this model includes holistic man and environment, health and self care. Holism is viewed in this model as concern for all component parts, or the composite of man functioning biologically, symbolically, and socially. Health is a reflection of the integrity of the whole. *Social space* as viewed within this conceptual model is the nursing system appropriate for the meeting of self care demand within agency as mandated by society. The systems from which the nurse may select include the wholly compensatory, the partially compensatory, and the supportive-educative systems. The *substantive focus* of this model is the concept of self care in its various forms. Self care needs are both universal and health deviating; self care agency is shared by the responsible adult with members of the health care system when self care demand exceeds self care capacity.

The Roy Adaptation Model

Some of the major concepts included in Roy's model are man-environment, health illness continuum, and adaptation. Holistic man's position on the health illness continuum is a function of his positive or negative responses to the changing environment, his adaptation or maladaptation. Nursing aims to promote the positive adaptative responses. Modes of adaptation identified by Roy include: physiologic needs, self concept, role function, and interdependence. Each of these modes may act as a focal, contextual, or residual stimulus for each other mode. Adaptive modes are considered intervening variables between needs and behavior. Roy further describes the adaptation response (positive) as occurring in an adaptation level zone. Adaptation problems occur with inadequate responses to need deficits or excesses. The adaptive mechanisms of regulator and cognator are mediators between the stimuli and behavioral response. The defined goal of nursing is to promote man's adaptation in each of the adaptive modes in situations of health and illness. Nursing activities include observation of man's behavior in the adaptive modes with identification of focal, contextual, and residual stimuli, diagnosis of an adaptation problem, and selection of methods to alter or remove the stimuli precipitating the problem (Roy 1971, 1974, 1976).

In summary, an analysis of the interrelationships posited in the theory yields the following propositional statements:

1. Holistic man is a biopsychosocial being, in constant interaction with a changing environment, who has health and illness as one dimension of his life.

2. The nature of man's interaction with the internal and external environment is a response to changes in the environment directed towards the maintenance of his biopsychosocial integrity.

3. To respond positively and adapt to his changing environment, man uses innate and acquired mechanisms.

4. Man adapts in response to the focal, contextual, and residual stimuli to which he is exposed, and the combined effects of these stimuli determine his adaptation level.

5. The stimuli must be within the zone of man's adaptation level to achieve a positive response.

6. Stimuli outside man's adaptive level lead to a maladaptive response and to adaptation problems.

7. Man has two adaptive mechanisms, regulator and cognator, that mediate his responses to needs.

8. Man's needs are expressed as behavior through four adaptive modes: physiologic, self concept, role function, and interdependence.

9. Focal, contextual, and residual stimuli may be identified for each adaptive mode and for each adaption problem.

10. Nurses assess man's adaptive and maladaptive behaviors in each of his four adaptive modes in relation to the different types of stimuli and the regulator and cognator adaptive mechanisms.

The model appears to stress relativity to a greater extent than universality, and reductionism more than emergence. However, described by Roy as a systems theory, this seems to present some inconsistency. The degree of openness seen in this model is most compatible with those systems theorists who view health as open and illness as the closing of the system.

Roy views man as a biopsychosocial being, in constant interaction with the environment. A major focus in this model, adaptation, is directed toward the maintenance of his biopsychosocial integrity. The emphasis on adaptation gives rise to expectation of influence of the external locus of developmental change. The *social space* defined within this framework is perhaps best represented by the concepts of focal, contextual, and residual stimuli.

The *substantive focus* for this model may be described as the two adaptive mechanisms, the cognator and regulator, that mediate his response to needs. Man's needs are expressed through four adaptive modes: physiologic, self concept, role function, and independence.

INTERRELATIONSHIPS AMONG NURSING THEORY, RESEARCH, EDUCATION, AND PROFESSIONAL PRACTICE

The scientific discipline and the professional practice of nursing have been best described as emergent. Evolutionary change within the past half century has been rapidly accelerating as new knowledge is discovered, broad under-standings are developed, scientific investigations are frequent, and pro-fessional practice is enhanced and modified by the knowledge base developed. In a comprehensive review of the emerging patterns of nursing research, Schlotfeldt (1977) and Gortner and Nahm (1977) trace the historical progression of nursing research and education from attention to the studies of nursing, nursing education, and nursing students to the more recent focus on clinical research, i.e., patient care research.

Nursing leaders have, more noticeably in the past 20 years, com-municated the need for the development of the science of nursing, including integration of components of theory, research, education, and practice (Johnson 1974, Downs 1969, Jacox 1974, Gortner 1975). Concomitantly, there have been demonstrated attempts at such inte-gration.

The conceptual frameworks of King (1971), Rogers (1970), Orem, (1971), and Roy (1976) have been utilized in the development of educa-tional programs for professional practitioners. Each of these theorists presents substantial data, particularly drawn from observations of nurs-ing practice situations, and theoretical arguments, particularly drawn from basic and behavioral sciences, in support of the developed con-ceptual models. The manner in which the conceptualizations and data are organized justifies the models as relevant to the science and prac-tice of nursing.

These conceptual frameworks provide the basis for the substantive analyses included in the chapters that follow. Particular attention will be directed toward the exploration of inconsistencies between these conceptual frameworks and the psychiatric mental health theories.

References

Aldous J: Strategies for developing family theory. J Marriage and the Family 32:250–257, 1970

Downs FS: Some critical issues in nursing research. Nurs Forum 8:392–404, 1969

Fawcett J: The "what" of theory development. In Theory Development: What, Why, How?, New York, National League for Nursing, 1978, p. 26

Fawcett J: A framework for analysis and evaluation of conceptual models of nursing. Nurse Educator, Nov.-Dec.:10–14, 1980

Fitzpatrick JJ: Patients' perception of time: current research. Int Nurs Rev, 27:148–153, 1980

Gortner SR: Research for the practice profession. Nurs Res, 24:193–197, 1975

Gortner SR, Nahm H: An overview of nursing research in the United States. Nurs Res, 26:10–33, 1977

Hill R, Mattessich P: Family development theory and lifespan development. In Baltes, P, Brimm O: Lifespan Development and Behavior, Vol. II. New York, Academic Press, 1979, 162–200

Hultsch D, Plemons J: Life events and life span development. In Baltes P, Brimm O (Eds).: Life Span Development and Behavior, New York, Academic Press, 1979

Jacox A: Nursing research and the clinician. Nurs Outlook, 22:382–385, 1974

Johnson DE: Development of theory: a requisite for nursing as a primary health profession. Nurs Res, 28:372–377, 1974

Kaufman A: Time, stress, perception model for theory development. In Norris M (Ed.): Proc First Nurs Theory Conf, Univ of Kansas Medical Center, Dept of Nursing Education, March, 1969

King IM: Conceptual frame of reference for nursing. Nurs Res, 17:27–31, 1968

King IM: Toward a Theory for Nursing, New York, John Wiley & Sons, 1971

Maruyama M: The second cybernetics: deviation amplifying mutual causal processes. Am Scient, 51:164–179, 1963

Miller JG: Living systems: basic concepts. In Gray W, Duhl F, Rizzo N (Eds.): General Systems Theory and Psychiatry, Boston, Little, Brown & Co., 1969

Muller TG: The Nature and Direction of Psychiatric Nursing, Philadelphia, J. B. Lippincott Co., 1950

Nursing Development Conference Group. Concept Formalization in Nursing: Process and Product, Boston, Little, Brown & Co., 1973

Nye FI, Berardo FM: Emerging Conceptual Frameworks in Family Analysis, New York, Macmillan Co., 1966

Orem DE: Nursing: Concepts of Practice, New York, McGraw-Hill, 1971

Peplau HE: Interpersonal Relations in Nursing, New York, G. P. Putnam's Sons, 1952

Rogers ME: An Introduction to the Theoretical Basis of Nursing, Philadelphia, F. A. Davis, 1970

Rogers ME: Nursing, a science of unitary man. In Riehl J, Roy C: Conceptual Models for Nursing Practice, 2nd ed. New York, Appleton-Century-Crofts, 1980

Roy C: Adaptation: a basis for nursing practice. Nurs Outlook, 19:254–257, 1971

Roy C: The Roy adaptation model. In Riehl JP, Roy C (Eds.): Conceptual Models for Nursing Practice, New York, Appleton-Century-Crofts, 1974

Roy C: Introduction to Nursing: An Adaptation Model, Englewood Cliffs, New Jersey, Prentice-Hall, 1976

Schlotfeldt RM: Nursing research: reflection of values. Nurs Res, 26:4–9, 1977

Sills GM: Research in the field of psychiatric nursing, 1952-1977. Nurs Res, 26:201–207, 1977

Sills GM: Hildegard E. Peplau: leader, practitioner, academician, scholar, and theorist. Perspect Psychiatr Care, 16:122–128, 1978

Tudor G: Sociopsychiatric nursing approach to intervention in a problem of mutual withdrawal on a mental hospital ward. Psychiatry, 15:193–217, 1952

von Bertalanffy L: General systems theory and psychiatry: an overview. *In* Gray W, Duhl F, Rizzo N (Eds): General Systems Theory and Psychiatry, Boston, Little Brown & Co, 1969

Whall A: Congruence between existing theories of family functioning and nursing theories. Adv Nurs Sci, 3:59–67, 1980

2 THE CRISIS PERSPECTIVE: RELATIONSHIP TO NURSING

Joyce J. Fitzpatrick

Although the term "crisis theory" is commonly used, there is also attention in the literature to crisis as a perspective for scientific inquiry rather than as characterized by the more formal attributes of theory. The crisis perspective has been proposed as a framework for conceptualizing human behavior. Several concepts inherent in this crisis perspective make it especially attractive to nursing, e.g., stress, equilibrium, change, health. These same concepts are intimately linked to a nursing perspective. As such, it has been widely adopted and acclaimed within the nursing literature, often without the theoretical reformulation necessary for a nursing perspective.

This presentation will first examine the major historical theoretical developments in the crisis literature, with particular attention to the significant contributions within the discipline of nursing. Major theoretical propositions within the crisis perspective will be identified and discussed in relation to the concepts of person, environment, health, and nursing, concepts that are proposed as essential to conceptual delineations within the discipline of nursing. Analysis and evaluation of the consistency between the crisis model and extant nursing models will be focused on the identification of necessary reformulations of the crisis perspective. Such theoretical reformulations will be discussed in terms of their resultant implications for nursing professional practice, education, and research.

HISTORICAL
DEVELOPMENTS   Lindemann's (1944) classic presentation of grief reactions following the Coconut Grove fire in Boston is widely accepted as the beginning point of the focus on crisis as a way of understanding human experiences. During the years that followed, Erich Lindemann and Gerald Caplan, in their association together at the Harvard School of Public Health, further developed the crisis perspective. Caplan more formally developed the theory, and is credited as the founder of the crisis theory perspective. His presentation of

this perspective is described in detail in *An Approach to Community Mental Health*, (1961) and *Principles of Preventative Psychiatry* (1964).

Because of the psychoanalytic and psychiatric orientation of the pioneers in this area, crisis theory is often linked to a psychodynamic perspective. As will be discussed, however, Caplan, Lindemann, and Rappaport attempted to move away from the psychoanalytic model. Ego psychologists Allport, Erikson, and Maslow, whose perspectives are focused on the normal person's life experiences with growth and development, have also contributed theory which has molded the crisis perspective, particularly in terms of the descriptions of maturational crisis. Exploration of Erikson's model will be included in this chapter, as an example of the ego psychologists' approach.

Significant sociological factors influenced the development of the crisis theory perspective. During World War II and the Korean War a "front lines" method of intervention was used for treatment of military persons experiencing stress. Glass (1957) describes the crisis intervention techniques that were used. From his observations of sociocultural transition states in the 1940's and 1950's, ranging from migration to natural disaster, Tyhurst (1957) presents an even broader perspective of crisis. The social and cultural transition states described by Tyhurst are often understood as precipitating situational crises. The 1961 Report of the Joint Commission on Mental Illness and Health in the United States, published in *Action for Mental Health*, had a significant influence on the development of crisis intervention as a treatment modality. This further enhanced the theoretical development of the crisis perspective. The Community Mental Health Centers Act, federal legislation enacted in 1963, provided funding for the development of community based programs for the delivery of mental health services. There were five essential components of a community mental health center that were necessary to qualify for federal funds. Significant to the crisis movement was the inclusion of emergency mental health services as one of these five essential components. Crisis intervention services became the frequently utilized treatment modality for delivery of emergency mental health services. Despite the present decline in the community mental health movement, crisis intervention services continue to be offered, accompanied by a variety of formal and informal supporting social structures, e.g., health care agencies. An additional significant movement, that of suicide prevention, developed along with the community mental health and crisis intervention movements. This suicide prevention movement, since historically linked to crisis intervention, often has conceptual ties which are similarly linked to the crisis perspective. For example, a suicidal crisis is often offered as an example of a mental health state that necessitates intervention.

The most significant application of crisis theory and crisis intervention methodology to the discipline of nursing is the text developed by Aguilera, Messick, and Farrell (1970). This text and its 1974 and 1978 revisions provide the basis for much of the basic educational and professional practice dimensions of the current nursing focus on the crisis theory perspective. More recent contributions to the crisis perspective from the discipline of nursing include the work of Hall and Weaver (1974) and Hoff (1978). At the present time almost all major psychiatric mental health nursing texts include some attention to crisis theory and crisis intervention as a treatment modality. Additional evidence of the conceptual congruence between the nursing and crisis perspectives is supported by reference to crisis theory and intervention in the other clinical subspecialties in nursing. Some educational programs, in fact, include crisis intervention as a clinical subspecialty, rather than the more traditional areas of concern.

Theoretical Components

The conceptualizations of Lindemann, Caplan, and Erikson are presented for the relevance to the crisis theory perspective. The same clinical situation is related to each of these conceptualizations in order to more clearly explicate the theoretical components inherent in the particular conceptualization. The clinical situation to be described within each of the selected conceptualizations is that of a seventeen-year-old male who presents himself to a walk-in crisis center, reporting difficulty sleeping, general fatigue, inability to concentrate, and suicidal thoughts. The adolescent reports that, 2 months previously, he experienced the death of his father. This particular example is not an unusual occurrence in the mental health field. Although some specifics of this situation will be given attention in the discussion of theoretical perspectives of crisis, an attempt will also be made to relate the conceptualizations to a more general clinical view.

Lindemann's Perspective

Lindemann described the psychological and somatic symptomatology that occurs in response to a loss. Manifestations of the grief reaction may be observed immediately following the crisis or they may be delayed. Extreme reactions or the absence of grieving in response to a loss are proposed by Lindemann to be abnormal.

Lindemann's description of the symptomatology includes attention to sighing respirations, reports of fatigue, a change in the sensorium, feelings of guilt, a loss of warmth in interpersonal relationships, anger, and hostility. Distortions or exaggerations in the grief reactions may be characterized by a more profound display of these symptoms. Although Lindemann mentions the concept anticipatory grief, he does not place much emphasis on its development or therapeutic value.

Lindemann advocates mental health intervention to assist individuals to deal with their grief reactions.

Based on Lindemann's conceptualization of grief reactions, the intervention in the clinical situation of the suicidal adolescent male would be focused on assisting the individual to move through the normal stages of grieving. The symptomatology that is presented would be understood to be normally characteristic of grieving or bereavement. Intervention would be aimed toward detailed assessment of the characteristics of the grieving process to ascertain whether there is normal movement through the process or whether there is some pathological process, such as the acquisition of symptoms belonging to the last illness of the deceased, or the expression of furious hostility toward specific persons, e.g., the physician who cared for his terminally ill father. The essential focus of therapeutic intervention would be the sharing of grief work with the young man, to assist him to find new patterns of rewarding interaction. Comfort through rituals, e.g., religious ceremonies, would be encouraged. The primary goal of intervention would be for the young male to understand his sense of loss, and develop an acceptable formulation of his future relationship to his deceased father.

Within Lindemann's conceptualization, particular attention might be focused on the suicidal ideation as related to some category of mental illness. The most congruous interpretation would be a psychoanalytic perspective on suicide, e.g., the understanding of anger turned inward.

Erikson's Perspective

Erikson proposed a developmental model derived from the psychoanalytic perspective, i.e., within the model there are definite conceptual links to the psychoanalytic perspective. Each of the developmental stages included in the model are also referred to by Erikson as a crisis. He considers these stages as opportunities for individuals to increase both personal and social organization.

Erikson's description and elaboration of development included attention to eight stages. These include (1) basic trust versus basic mistrust (oral sensory); (2) autonomy vs. shame and doubt (muscular anal); (3) initiative vs. guilt (locomotive genital); (4) industry vs. inferiority (latency); (5) identity vs. role confusion (puberty and adolescence); (6) intimacy vs. isolation (young adulthood); (7) generativity vs. stagnation (adulthood); and (8) ego integrity vs. despair (maturity). The emphasis is on the childhood stages with some minor attention to stages of adult development.

There is the underlying assumption within Erikson's model that individuals develop a personality according to these predetermined stages which represent steps in the process. Erikson also proposed that society is structured to deal with individuals as they develop through these stages. In a sense, there is an expectation of a process of development that serves to maintain the social order.

As a treatment modality, Erikson proposes psychoanalysis which is most consistent with his model. His presentation of dimensions of the analyst's role included attention to cure-research, objectivity-participation, knowledge-imagination, and tolerance-indignation. The therapist is therefore described not only as a professional but also as a scientist.

Applying Erikson's conceptualization to the clinical example of the adolescent male who is suicidal, one would attend to two basic levels of personality structure, viz., the level of organization and interaction of id, ego, and superego, and the level of developmental stage. The goal of therapy would be to help the individual resolve the conflict and continue to develop through the psychosocial stages.

Interpretations of behavior would necessarily be related to these components of personality and the levels of functioning. For example, one could conclude that there is a degree of self reproach evidenced that reflects a strong superego or conscience. The ego's responsibility is to maintain the inner order on which the outer order depends. In this situation there might be considered neither inner nor outer order, in that the ego defenses are not strong enough to tide the adolescent through the loss of his father. This death may evoke in the adolescent some of the early experiences of the stage of initiative vs. guilt. The adolescent may understand himself as partially responsible for the death of his father and thus experience again the early childhood conflict centered around sexual rivalry with his father.

As with Lindemann's conceptualization, there would be some focus on understanding the suicidal behavior as anger turned inward. Thus therapeutic attempts would be directed toward methods of identifying and understanding this anger and channeling it into more constructive behaviors.

Caplan's Perspective

Caplan focuses most directly on the elaboration of the crisis perspective per se. He proposed that peak periods or sudden turning points could be identified within the human experience. Characteristic of such periods are both a rise in tension and a mobilization of resources. According to Caplan, a crisis is by definition a period of disequilibrium which presents a threat to the individual's homeostasis. In periods where crises are not present, there can be identified and described both intrapsychic and interpersonal mechanisms to maintain equilibrium.

During a crisis an individual is confronted with a problem that is of basic importance to him, yet cannot be easily solved by his normally useful problem solving mechanisms. This presenting problem is directly related to the individual's instinctual needs. Caplan describes the development of a crisis according to four phases. During the first phase some threat to the system equilibrium is presented. During this period there is an initial rise in the anxiety level as the person recognizes and, at times, acknowledges the threat present, and the imbalance between internal needs and resources and external demands. In the second phase the individual's usual problem solving abilities are unsuccessful in meeting the current challenge. Thus, again some increase in anxiety occurs. In the third phase, with even more anxiety present, the individual uses every resource available. At the same time that the individual is using usual intrapsychic resources, he or she is seeking new resources from the environment. There is an attempt to find new ways to solve the problem. During the fourth phase the anxiety is at an intolerable level, the problem is not resolved, and the individual has exhausted the known intrapersonal and interpersonal resources to solve the problem.

Within this framework is not only a focus on previous learning that has occurred in problem solving abilities but also a focus on present patterns of behaving. Since the period of disorganization characteristic of a crisis generates attention to previous conflicts, particularly those symbolically linked with the present problem, there is an attempt to integrate the past with present experiencing.

Caplan proposes that the state of maturity and the structure of the ego are important dimensions of mental health. Assessment of mental health status therefore is focused on the individual's ability to withstand stress and anxiety and thus maintain equilibrium, the degree of reality recognized in solving problems, and the repertoire of coping mechanisms available to the individual (Caplan 1961).

In the clinical example cited, i.e., that of the adolescent suicidal male, there would be an assessment process focused on identification of need response patterns, problem solving mechanisms, and intrapsychic description of the suicidal adolescent. Clearly the present experience would be understood as a crisis, i.e., not only the death of his father, but also the adolescent's response to this experience. Symbolic links with previous conflicts not unlike that proposed through Erikson's model would be identified as part of the assessment. The individual would be assisted in understanding his present thoughts, feelings, and behaviors in light of both past experiences and present reality. Levels of anxiety and disequilibrium would be identified. Therapeutic intervention would be focused on assisting the adolescent to learn new problem solving skills by developing an awareness and understanding of the present experience. Additionally, emphasis in the intervention process would be placed on a long range perspective on the person's mental health.

SUMMARY OF THE CRISIS
PERSPECTIVE   Several propositional statements, based primarily on the explications of Caplan, can be used to summarize the crisis perspectives. These include:

1. The life process includes a succession of crisis experiences.
2. A crisis poses a threat to the individual which places equilibrium and sense of self in jeopardy.
3. The goal of crisis resolution is the return to the pre-crisis level of functioning, i.e., the restoration of equilibrium.
4. Crises possess the potential for opportunity, i.e., they can be growth experiences.
5. A crisis is by definition time limited; as such it is a transitional point in the person's experience of life.
6. Specific phases of the crisis experience can be identified and described.
7. Crises are more accessible to intervention at their peak.
8. Precipitating events may be identified in relation to the occurrence of crises.
9. Previous experiences with crises increase the ability to function in current crises.
10. The crisis experience includes a constellation of feelings associated with the upset state.
11. Resolution of crises may be directly linked to mental health and illness; crises may be resolved in positive or negative ways.

NURSING'S APPLICATION OF THE
CRISIS PERSPECTIVE   Crisis intervention theory has been developed from the overall crisis perspective. Consistent with this development of theory, professionals, particularly those in the mental health field, have attempted to more systematically articulate the theoretical rationale underlying their intervention modalities. During the 1970's, there was a recognition of a need for inclusion of both the crisis perspective and the crisis intervention framework into the science, education, and professional practice of nursing.

Hall and Weaver's (1974) approach to relating the crisis perspective to nursing intervention is direct. These authors clearly state their goal as the application of the concepts within crisis intervention theory to nursing care. They have broadened the applicability to all of nursing practice rather than restricting it to those who intervene primarily with persons with a mental illness. Hall and Weaver also present a broad spectrum of examples related to the crisis perspective. They also deal with both maturational and situational crises.

Hoff's (1978) presentation on the nature of crisis and the application of crisis intervention techniques in helping individuals experiencing crises is an even broader perspective. Crisis intervention is presented in a manner useful to all health professionals and human service workers. In addition, Hoff adds an important dimension in her special focus on suicidal crises.

Aguilera, Messick, and Farrell (1970)[2] presented a brief, yet inclusive, text on crisis intervention, focused particularly on crisis intervention methodology and its usefulness in nursing practice. In developing their framework for client assessment and intervention, these authors make some comparisons to other psychotherapeutic modalities, viz., psychoanalysis and brief psychotherapy. They then translate the crisis intervention modality into a problem solving approach. It is assumed that this emphasis on problem solving may be directly linked to the concomitant emphasis within the larger scientific nursing community. Frequently the nursing process has been described as a problem solving process. Within this problem solving perspective, both crisis intervention and nursing intervention can be viewed as a logical sequence of behaviors that is aimed at goal achievement and problem resolution.

A basic paradigm of crisis is presented by Aguilera and Messick. This paradigm, as developed, includes attention to the major propositional statements previously presented as a summary of the crisis perspective. The primary contributions of Aguilera et al. seem to be in their application to nursing situations and their design of an uncomplicated model which is useful across crisis situations. The conceptual approach is focused on the concepts of crisis: equilibrium, perception, balancing factors, coping mechanisms, and situational supports. They present various descriptions of both situational and maturational crises which serve to illustrate the relationships among the basic concepts they identify, and more significantly the relationships of these concepts to the manifestations of crisis. Since these authors are primarily concerned with intervention modalities, much of the emphasis is on the professional practice dimension.

Within this crisis intervention model very little attention is paid to health as a central concept. There is no clear elaboration of the relationships between crisis and mental health and illness, but, as with the overall crisis perspective, there is a focus on prevention of mental illness through therapeutic intervention in crisis situations.

In relation to the clinical example of the adolescent suicidal male, Aguilera and Messick would attend to recognition of the precipitating factors that have led to the crisis and therefore, the state of disequilibrium. Using their paradigm, focus would be on assessment of the balancing factors present and absent. This particular crisis would be understood as related to the recent loss of the father, and the intervener would explore the anxiety and/or depression associated with that loss,

[2] The latest revision of this appears as Aguilera, DC and Messick, JM, *Crisis Intervention: Theory and Methodology*, 3rd edition, St. Louis: C. V. Mosby, 1978.

is intervention modalities there is specific focus on the pre-
mental illness and thus, the promotion of mental health.
intervention as a therapeutic modality for assisting individ-
lies, groups, and communities has been understood as theo-
nd experientially compatible with nursing interventions. The
nterventions are necessitated with persons experiencing nor-
lopmental events makes the use of the crisis intervention
rticularly appealing in professional nursing practice. Nursing
inherent in the nursing process, e.g., assessment and evalua-
also primary in crisis intervention techniques.

preceding discussion identifies some general considerations of
environment, health, and nursing within the crisis perspective.
attention is given to the proposed relationships within the crisis
toward the goal of explicating congruence between the crisis
rsing perspectives.

ecific nursing conceptualizations that are addressed in this sec-
clude those of Roy, King, and Orem. Reformulation of crisis
Rogers' nursing perspective is then presented, as this is viewed as
ovative scientific approach which will enhance the further devel-
t of the discipline of nursing.

GRUENCE BETWEEN CRISIS PERSPECTIVE
NURSING MODELS
The description of persons within
risis perspective is particularly consistent with the adaptation
l proposed by Roy (1976). Roy's description of person as a bio-
osocial being permits attention to the psychological and physio-
al dimensions included within the equilibrium aspects of the crisis
els. According to Roy, a person's position on the health-illness
inuum is related to responses to changes in the environment.
se human responses may be characterized as adaptation or
adaptation. Need deficits or excesses can be described as manifesta-
s of maladaptation. This understanding of the health-illness con-
um presented by Roy is consistent with a medical model crisis
spective such that excesses or deficits would be labeled as mental
ess. The delayed or exaggerated grief responses described by
demann would be examples of maladaptation described by Roy.

Roy's model further proposes that persons use innate and acquired
echanisms to adapt, and that persons have some level of adaptation.
his again is consistent with the crisis focus on personality characteris-
s or capabilities for responding to crisis, and with the understanding
at persons possess coping skills which are used in determining their
ovement through the crisis experience. Roy's description of the four
daptive modes, physiological, self concept, interdependence, and role

and would assess the previous and current coping skills. For example,
the young male might be assisted to understand this loss in relation to
other experienced crises.

Aguilera and Messick, in discussing the theoretical aspects of
suicide, propose that, while there might be multiple causes, "suicidal
behavior can usually be related to three primary motivations: loss of
communication, ambivalence about life and death, and the effects of
suicidal behavior on significant others" (1978, p. 111). Thus, it is likely
that intervention based on this model also would directly focus on these
aspects. The communication of the young male would be understood
as including messages about hopelessness and helplessness related to
the loss of the father. The intervener may understand the communication to be directed to the father or to another significant person in the
adolescent's world. The ambivalence characteristic of all suicidal behavior would be assumed to be present, and would be explored within
the intervention process. The intervener also would focus on assisting
the adolescent male to understand his communication patterns, and to
attempt to identify the significant other, perhaps mother, to whom the
young male desires to direct communication.

Aguilera and Messick briefly attend to the knowledge developed in
the field of suicidology and discuss a plan of assessment of suicide
potential that the therapist uses when there is suicidal communication.
Thus in this example, on initial contact, the therapist would assess the
suicide potential by gathering information about age and sex, suicidal
plan, symptoms, resources, communications, and significant others.
There is no direct, detailed explanation of how this information would
be used in the therapeutic situation. The goal, however, is to prevent
the suicide.

REVIEW OF EXISTING REFORMULATIONS
OF CRISIS THEORY
The conceptual reformulations of crisis
theory proposed by Taplin (1971) and Narayan and Joslin (1980) are
relevant. They share the characteristic of arguing against the medical
model focus of illness which is inherent in the psychiatric views proposed by Lindemann and Caplan.

Taplin (1971) proposes a cognitive perspective that includes attention to perceptual and learning processes. This cognitive perspective is
presented as a useful means of guiding systematic inquiry, e.g., by an
approach to defining crisis in terms of specific personality variables. In
addition, crisis is distinguished from stress, qualitatively, and from critical periods or developmental milestones by means of assessment of
behavioral functioning. Taplin also suggests that the cognitive perspective yields new avenues of approach to crisis intervention. Examples of

particular intervention strategies that would be used include the teaching of information processing techniques, e.g., information assimilation, the use of social rites and practices which legitimize temporary disorganization, the teaching of basic mastery skills necessary for role performance in society, and teaching of general life performance techniques. Taplin argues that the focus within the crisis perspective on homeostasis and psychoanalysis is neither heuristic nor pragmatic as a theoretical approach. He suggests that the cognitive perspective is a less well integrated theoretical framework, which in itself may be understood as either advantageous or disadvantageous, depending on the definitions of theory and uses of theory to which one subscribes.

Based on Taplin's conceptualization, the clinical situation of the adolescent suicidal male used as an example clearly would be labeled a crisis. Taplin would suggest that the behavioral functioning, in this case some inability to function as compared to previously, would be essential to the assessment process. Specific interventions might be focused on assisting the young male to focus on life performance techniques. For example, it is conceivable that the young male will assume some of the family responsibilities previously belonging to his father. Mastery of new skills would be a desired outcome. The young male would be encouraged to make use of ritualistic activities to provide some present structure and organization.

Undoubtedly, some attempt would be made to understand the suicidal behavior in terms of specific personality characteristics. The individual would be understood as having experienced a psychological "overload," i.e., the information to be handled as a result of this new experience overwhelms the perceptual field. Intervention would be focused on changing the cognitive patterns such that the individual learns new ways of coping with his new environment.

Narayan and Joslin (1980) proposed a holistic nursing model of crisis as an alternative to the medical model perspective inherent in much of the crisis literature. Basic concepts within this nursing model are growth and self care. While the authors move away from discussion of mental illness as a result of poorly resolved crises, they instead focus on a state of depleted health potential, viewed as part of the health continuum. Within this health state is an alteration in the functioning pattern, which leads to some loss of resources.

Within the Narayan and Joslin conceptualization the clinical situation of the adolescent suicidal male would be viewed as an opportunity for growth and self-enhancement. The young male would be assisted to learn more about himself through the experience of his father's death. Focus in assessment would be on the alterations in his patterns of functioning and the experienced loss of father as a resource.

Because of the suicidal ideation, the individual may be understood

to be in the peak of crisis or the flounde
ing, where there is too much conflictin
cognitive understanding of the crisis ex
and Joslin is not unlike that proposed b
would be to help the individual process
learning new patterns of cognitive funct
tential would lead to death. One might
there is some diminished energy available,
health potential.

RELATIONSHIP OF CRISIS PERSPE
TO BASIC NURSING CONCEPTS
be understood as including a range of ess
extent to which the crisis perspective include
based on the discipline of nursing is of particu
perspective will be discussed in terms of the
of person, environment, health, and nursing.

Delineations within the crisis perspective
characteristics of persons. Individuals are pe
threshold for coping with stresses that is formed
is described as, personality. Previous experien
about, crises shape the individual's personality,
the experience of the present crisis. The primal
behaviors of individuals in crisis is to assist in re
balance, the equilibrium, that is understood as
healthy state. Within this attempt at restoration, th
uses intrapersonal resources, e.g., coping skills
ences, but also relies upon interpersonal skills in
others in the environment.

Characteristics of environment attended to
perspective include the situational factors which
cipitating event and the interpersonal resources
available to the individual in crisis. Based on the dev
proposed by Erikson, various psychosocial events
stood as precipitating crises, e.g., adolescence, mar
though there is attention in the literature to the
situational and maturational crises, descriptive chara
individual's crisis experience are similar across these cat
the precipitating situational event accounts for this cat

Characteristics of the concept of health within the
tive are related to the positive or negative outcomes of c
Crisis theory, in its attention to equilibrium, stress, and
has links to the physiological perspective. Additionally, i

function, is also related to the crisis perspective. These adaptive modes can be understood as comparable to the exploration of coping behaviors; some changes in these components of the person are necessary in order to restore the equilibrium, or to adapt. Problems inherent within these dimensions can lead to difficulty resolving the crisis or difficulty in adapting.

Consistency between Roy's adaptation model and the cognitive model of crisis can be identified. Roy describes regulator and cognator adaptive mechanisms that mediate responses to needs not dissimilar from the cognitive processing proposed by Taplin. For example, the behavior expressed, according to Roy, through the role function adaptive mode may be understood as similar to the role mastery concept inherent in a cognitive crisis approach. Roy's attention to the adaptive modes is most consistent here. External stimuli are responsible for the changes experienced by the individual through the adaptive modes. Roy describes the nature of those stimuli as either focal, contextual, or residual. Thus, there is the opportunity for a range of individual responses depending on the combinations of type of stimuli, adaptive modes, and adaptive mechanisms.

Based on Roy's conceptual framework, intervention with the adolescent male in the clinical example cited would be initially focused on assessment of the adaptive mode where the problem occurs and identification of the environmental factors that are acting as stimuli. In the case of this suicidal male, one might identify a need deficit or maladaptation within the self concept mode, as the individual may experience his father's loss as a threat to his own identity. Changes in the environment would be structured in the intervention process so as to activate some change in the individual's adaptive mechanisms, and thus to facilitate adaptation. The adolescent male would be encouraged to use his innate and acquired mechanisms to adapt. The interpretation could be made that some emphasis might be placed on the cognator mechanism in this situation, since there is an intense need for the adolescent to develop an understanding of the situation.

King's system model of persons also describes a biopsychosocial organism interacting with both internal and external environments. Basic concepts within King's nursing perspective include perception, health, interpersonal relations, and social systems, where perception and health are characteristics of persons. This elaboration of the perceptual dimension of human functioning is most consistent with the cognitive conceptualization of crisis proposed by Taplin. Aspects of King's conceptual framework are also consistent with the more general crisis perspective. For example, the social system concept described by King could be understood similarly as social supports and resources within the crisis perspective.

King's model of nursing intervention is especially congruent with crisis intervention methodology. King proposes a process of action, reaction, interaction, and transaction that the nurse would use to assist individuals to achieve health. The process is focused on altering the individual's perception and cognition of the experience and the interaction with internal and external environments. For example, in the clinical example cited, there would be considerable attention to the development of a relationship that would lead to perceptual and cognitive awareness of the situation. The adolescent male would be helped to see how his perceptions and understandings are related to the loss of his father. The transaction level of intervention would be achieved when the therapist and the individual engaged in mutual goal setting to resolve the suicidal crisis. The mutual goal setting could be around various relevant areas, e.g., further enhancement of communication patterns, expression of aggression, and development of new coping skills. The primary emphasis of the intervention process would be to increase the level of health and, in this specific case, to resolve the crisis (King 1971).

Concepts basic to Orem's (1971) framework include persons, health, and self care, with particular emphasis on the self care dimension of human functioning. Orem describes persons as functioning biologically, symbolically, and socially. A person's position on the health-illness continuum is evidenced by behaviors related to cognition, biophysiological aspects, and social relationships. Persons have an innate need for self care that directs behaviors related to health.

Much consistency exists between the Orem self care model and the Roy adaptation model. It can be interpreted that Orem's conceptualization of nursing is, like Roy's, consistent with the psychiatric crisis perspective and with some components of the cognitive crisis perspective. An additional point of interest in Orem's model is the attention to symbolic human function. The emphasis on rituals as therapeutic processes within the crisis perspective is particularly appropriate here.

Orem describes universal and health deviation self care requirements that may be characteristic of any individual seeking assistance. The individual responds to these self care needs through self care agency, which might be understood as comparable to coping patterns or skills within the crisis perspective. In the clinical example cited, the adolescent male would be understood as having a self care agency deficit that requires professional intervention. The suicidal behavior would almost certainly be labeled as a deviation from health, and intervention would be focused on assessing the adolescent's self care demands.

In summary, there is some consistency between the crisis perspective and the conceptual frameworks of King, Orem, and Roy. Within each of these conceptualizations, primary attention is given to the concept of persons, with various definitions, descriptors, and subconcepts explicated. Environment is conceptualized as external, and somewhat opposing, to the individual, within the crisis perspective and in the conceptualizations included in the models of Roy, King, and Orem. Environment is of importance as a concept, but only achieves significance because of its influence on human behavior. Health as a concept is given more emphasis within the nursing models than within the crisis perspective. Clearly health is a goal defined within nursing, whereas crisis is less directly focused on this goal.

REFORMULATION OF CRISIS PERSPECTIVE AS RELATED TO ROGERS' CONCEPTUALIZATION

OF NURSING   Rogers proposes that the developmental process toward increasing complexity and diversity is characterized by wave patterns and rhythmic activity identifying the whole. The experience of human life is thus an experience of rhythms, with the characteristic peaks and troughs. Any dimension of the life process or the human experience can be viewed from this rhythm perspective.

While there is theoretical and empirical support for the rhythm component of Rogers' conceptualization, there have been no previous attempts to link this rhythm perspective to the crisis perspective. Some reformulations of the crisis perspective are necessary to achieve conceptual congruence. The basic concept that requires redefinition within the crisis perspective is equilibrium, which implies a balance or steady-state phenomenon. Because of the dynamic nonsteady nature of the human field described by Rogers, this equilibrium concept would necessarily be replaced by the concept of homeodynamics defining human and environmental patterns in a fluid, interacting way. Change in this basic definition of equilibrium or, more precisely, substitution of the concept homeodynamics, would not substantially alter the basic propositions inherent in the crisis perspective. The goal of the human system, and thus the goal of crisis intervention, would be changed to that of altering patterns within the human system so as to enhance the interaction with the environment. Health within Rogers' conceptual framework is manifestation of symphonic interaction of persons and their environments. Thus, congruency, consistency, and integrity characterize the rhythmic patterns that can be described.

Within this reformulation the rhythm term of "phase" would be more consistent than the "stage" so frequently used in developmental literature. One would then speak of the developmental phases of human experiencing. The crisis experiences would be conceptualized as the turning points in these developmental phases. Holistic manifestations of person environment interaction would necessarily be identified. These rhythms would be critical in describing not only the developmental phases but also the crisis experiences. Some holistic rhythmic patterns have been described as postulated indices of holistic persons. These include temporality, or nonlinear temporal rhythms, movement, consciousness, and perceptual experiences (Fitzpatrick 1980). The maturational crises that have been described in the crisis literature would then be examined for their similarities in terms of the manifestations of these holistic rhythmic patterns. More specifically, descriptions of the manifestations of temporal experience, for example, could be provided across crisis states. Most often individuals who are experiencing crises report a sense of present focus and time pressure.

Reformulations of the theoretical propositions within the crisis perspective provide an opportunity for integration of knowledge. This integration is particularly meaningful in the professional practice dimension of nursing.

IMPLICATIONS FOR RESEARCH, EDUCATION, AND PROFESSIONAL PRACTICE

Based on the integration of the crisis perspective and Rogers' conceptual framework, research on rhythmic manifestations of holistic human characteristics is a priority. The postulated indices of holistic persons previously identified, viz. temporality, movement, consciousness, and perceptual experiences, present concepts to conceptually and methodologically clarify. Programmatic research in some of these areas has already begun. A second avenue of research should focus on evaluation of the intervention modalities that are components of professional nursing practice derived from the conceptualizations.

Educational programs in nursing could use Rogers' conceptual framework for the curricula. Theoretical frameworks that would be integrated into learning experiences include the crisis theory perspective, the rhythm theory perspective, and the related derivations of these. Substantive knowledge generated through nursing research also would be mandated.

Professional nursing practice would be aimed at assisting individuals to change patterns of their human experience. Particular emphasis would be placed on assessments of the rhythm profiles of holistic indices. The interaction process would be used significantly to assist individuals to achieve their maximum health potential.

References

Action for Mental Health. Report of the Joint Commission on Mental Illness and Health. New York, Basic Books, 1961

Aguilera DC, Messick JM, Farrell J: Crisis Intervention: Theory and Methodology, St. Louis, C. B. Mosby, 1970

Aguilera DC, Messick JM: Crisis Intervention: Theory and Methodology (2nd ed.), St. Louis, C. V. Mosby, 1974

Aguilera DC, Messick JM: Crisis Intervention: Theory and Methodology (3rd ed.), St. Louis, C. V. Mosby, 1978

Caplan G: An Approach to Community Mental Health, New York, Grune and Stratton, 1961

Caplan G: Principles of Preventive Psychiatry, New York, Basic Books, Inc., 1964

Erikson EH: Childhood and Society (2nd ed.), New York, W. W. Norton and Company, 1963

Fitzpatrick JJ: Patients' perception of time: current research. Inter Nurs Rev, 27:148–153, 1980

Glass AT: Observations upon the epidemiology of mental illness in troops during warfare. Symposium on Preventive and Social Psychiatry. Walter Reed Army Institute of Research and The National Research Council, Washington, D.C., April 15–17, 1957.

Hall J, Weaver BA: Nursing of Families in Crisis, Philadelphia, J. B. Lippincott, 1974

Hoff LA: People in Crisis: Understanding and Helping, Menlo Park, CA, Addison Wesley, 1978

King IM: Toward a Theory for Nursing, New York, John Wiley & Sons, 1971

Lindemann E: Symptomatology and management of acute grief. Am J Psychiatry, 101:141–148, 1944

Narayan SM, Joslin DJ: Crisis theory and intervention: a critique of the medical model and proposal of a holistic nursing model. Adv Nurs Sci, 2:27–39, 1980

Orem DE: Nursing: Concepts of Practice, New York, McGraw Hill, 1971

Roy C: Introduction to Nursing: An Adaptation Model, Englewood Cliffs, New Jersey, Prentice-Hall, 1976

Taplin JR: Crisis theory: critique and reformulation. Community Ment Health J, 7:13–23, 1971

Tyhurst JS: The role of transition states—including disasters—in mental illness. Symposium on Preventive and Social Psychiatry. Walter Reed Army Institute of Research and the National Research Council, Washington, D.C., April 15-17, 1957

3 INDIVIDUAL PSYCHOTHERAPY: RELATIONSHIP OF THEORETICAL APPROACHES TO NURSING CONCEPTUAL MODELS

Ruth L. Johnston

The theoretical approaches addressed in this chapter are not presented as an exhaustive review of theories on which current psychiatric mental health practice is based. Rather, the approaches presented were selected to represent both the progress and problems inherent in the development of theory based practice. This cross-sectional view is designed to illustrate the changing emphasis from intrapsychic phenomena through interpsychic or interactional approaches, leading to an increasing emphasis on systems views. Included will be a presentation of the major psychiatric theories, the major nursing models, and the exploration of congruence between psychiatric theories and nursing models. Reformulation of theories needed for increased congruence will be identified.

Brief descriptions of psychoanalytic theory, modifications in this theory representative of interpersonal theory, and extensions included by Erikson as he developed his conceptualization of the eight-stage developmental process of man, are presented. Additionally, behavioral theory developing out of the work of Watson and Skinner within experimental psychology is recognized as a significantly different approach that has influenced a wide segment of practice, and also is included here. Some exploration of the impact of systems theories on individual approaches, and relating to communication and interaction theory is presented. Finally, Maslow's contributions to theory development and clinical practice are discussed.

Perhaps the most representative of current practice theoretical positions is an eclectic approach, selecting what appears to be best in various doctrines, methods, or styles. The eclectic approach presents serious problems to the development of a unified theory to guide practice, as does the grounded theory approach described by Aldous (1970). The selection of portions of theories, positions, and styles that appear best suited to the present situation offer a desired flexibility. This eclectic approach adds as a danger the increased likelihood of problems of logical inconsistency in both internal and external spheres. Additionally, problems inherent in comparisons through research are compounded by the different mix of ideas being tested. For these reasons, hypothesis testing and replication are limited. Development of new theories, and reformulation of old theories within the nursing perspective are recommended as viable alternatives to eclecticism. The clear articulation of valid nursing theories to guide psychiatric mental health practice is an identified need and major goal for the discipline.

The nursing models reviewed in this chapter include those of Peplau, Orem, King, Roy, and Rogers. Rather than explore the congruence-incongruence of each with each of the psychiatric mental health theories, some attempt at "best fit" will be undertaken. That is, those with identified existing congruence will be related with recommended reformulation to increase the relevance to and consistency with the nursing model. Behaviorism as interpreted for nursing by Loomis and Horsley (1974) will be related to other nursing models.

Among the strategies for theory development are these approaches: factor theory, grounded theory, borrowed theory, and conceptual frameworks (Aldous 1970). The discipline of nursing recently has been heavily involved in the development of conceptual frameworks. Reformulation of borrowed theory within those frameworks seems a most important and appropriate step in developing a theory based practice in psychiatric mental health nursing.

Paradigms that are useful in the evaluation of congruence between conceptual frameworks and borrowed theory include mechanistic, organismic, or relational (also called transactional, dialectical, or dynamic interactional). Issues related to these paradigms are identified by Hill and Mattessick (1979). Positions on these issues correlate with positions on openness of systems (Hultsch and Plemons 1979) as well as on the organismic versus mechanistic views of man.

External versus internal locus of developmental change involves man the actor (internal) or man as reactor (external) as the predominant stimulus for change. Reductionism versus emergence offers another comparative issue. The mechanistic model assumes that any behavioral skill can be reduced to a simpler, more elementary form (reductionism); while emergence implies that later forms cannot be reduced to earlier forms. Emergence is compatible with the organismic view. In the concept of emergence, the symbolic level of hierarchical order makes reductionism incompatible with systems theory. The conceptualization of emergence is consistent with unidirectionality, an additional issue, while bidirectionality is compatible with reductionism.

A fourth issue, universality versus relativity, provides for further comparison. The organismic view requires conceptualization of development as universal; individuals evolve through a common sequence of developmental stages. Relational or dialectic models are compatible with biologic universality but additionally accept culturally variant and genetic experiential uniqueness. Mechanistic or reactive models require relativity in development.

PSYCHIATRIC THEORIES OF FREUD, SULLIVAN, AND ERIKSON

Freudian Psychoanalysis

Within the psychoanalytic approach, the view of man posited by Freud and continuing throughout the development of this theoretical formulation is one of strong biological and genetic base. *Man* is viewed as a complex biological organism with an individual personality and recognized to be a member of a highly organized social group. Beginning with the conceptualization of man dominated by two instincts, Freud gradually moved to the structural theory of personality to explain the individual nature that develops within the complex biological organism.

It may be helpful to review the structures, systems, or centers of psychic functioning described by Freud. Freud's structural theory or model of psychic functioning evolved over a period of nearly three decades, with a more or less formalized presentation in *The Ego and the Id* (Freud 1960). The structural systems of this model were described by their mode of functioning and conditions of energy. As described, the mental apparatus is divided into three parts: id, ego, and superego. The id is the oldest of the mental processes or provinces. It is conceptualized to contain everything that is inherited, that is present at birth, that is fixed in the constitution, i.e., the instincts. The ego develops out of the cortical layer of the id, is adapted for the reception of external stimuli, and is thus in contact with the external world. The superego forms within the ego, incorporating or prolonging the influence of the parents through observation of the ego, and directs, corrects, and threatens punishments in the pattern of previous parental admonishments.

This theory includes three fundamental principles of the mental apparatus and of the behavior of living organisms. The first, the *principle of stability*, posits that the basic function of the mental apparatus consists of sustaining the homeostatic equilibrium within the organism. This equilibrium is continuously disturbed by the very process of life as well as by the changing environmental influences. Re-establishing homeostatic equilibrium is the major purpose of the ego. Ego functions include the perception of internal disturbances (needs, sensations, etc.), the sensory perception of the external situation upon which gratification of needs depends, and the integration of these perceptions.

The executive function, that of determining the behavioral response, follows the integration of internal and external perceptions. Additionally, the ego functions to protect the psyche from excessive external stimuli (Alexander 1961).

The second fundamental principle, the *principle of economy or inertia*, posits that "every organism is born with unconditioned reflexes useful for maintaining those constant conditions within the organism which are necessary for life" (Alexander 1961, p. 166). This principle is manifested in the development of the organism, through the stages of groping experimentation to ways of re-establishing equilibrium that are characterized by automatic, repetitious behaviors. This mechanism provides economy of energy advantageous to the organism. Not advantageous, however, is the loss of flexibility in response to changing conditions of growth, and changing environmental influences.

Third is the *principle of surplus energy*. Progression from birth to maturity is largely predetermined, a series of steps leading toward the mastery of functions that make the human being independent of parents. The dynamisms of fixation and regression mark this course to maturity; growth is biologically determined, fixation and regression represent the individual personality's resistance to the growth process. The energy not needed to maintain life is surplus energy, the source of all sexual activity. In summary, the life process in man is characterized by three phases, growth to maturation, the reproductive years, and the last phase, marked by the decline of function (Alexander 1961).

Since psychoanalytic theory is essentially intrapsychic in focus, less attention is given to *environment* and health. The biological nature of man limits environmental influence to the social context in which the individual aspect of personality is molded. Environment is discussed primarily as that highly organized social group.

Health is not made explicit within this theory. The implicit definition of health (the absence of pathology) that characterizes the medical model is relevant here. To attain health, one undertakes to resolve intrapsychic conflict and thus lessen the resulting pathology that may impinge upon the health of the individual.

Sullivan's Interpersonal Theory

The interpersonal theory of psychiatry of Sullivan (1953) represents a modification of psychoanalytic theory by recognition and addition of two major concepts. These include a shift in emphasis from intra- to interpsychic phenomena, and more extensive use of the developmental approach. Trained in psychoanalysis, Sullivan deviated from the observational approach of psychoanalytic methodology to a participant observer role, and clearly demonstrated a shift to an interpersonal approach in both theory and practice strategies. His interest in the problems of communication is apparent. The interpersonal theory is basically the psychiatric perspective on the study of interpersonal relations, or the operational approach a psychiatrist might make as a participant observer with individuals experiencing interpersonal conflict.

Sullivan proposes that a large part of mental disorder results from, and is perpetuated by, inadequate communication. Anxiety is proposed as the source of interference in the communication problems. Secondly, he proposes that each person in any two-person relationship is involved as a portion of an interpersonal field, rather than as a separate entity, in processes that affect and are affected by the field.

Acceptance of the psychoanalytic formulations of conscious and unconscious processes is apparent. Additionally, Sullivan reformulates developmental processes from the biologically dominated psychosexual development postulated by psychoanalysis to include the nature and impact of experience.

This impact of experience is elaborated further in the postulation of three modes of experience, the prototaxic, parataxic, and syntaxic. Prototaxic mode includes those experiences that are presymbolic, or prior to the development and use of symbols. The parataxic mode is described as the use of symbols in a private or autistic way, an individualistic mode. Finally, syntaxic mode is that manner through which one person can communicate experience to another, conceptualized in symbols that are defined in a similar way.

Also important to Sullivan's theory of child development is the concept of dynamism. Dynamisms involve the patterns of energy transformation that characterize the interpersonal relations that make up the distinctively unique human. The interpersonal field is made up of interaction of a variety of dynamisms of two or more individuals. Further elaboration posits two types of dynamisms: conjunctive, of which intimacy is an example, and disjunctive, involving anxiety and leading toward disintegration of the interpersonal situation. Conjunctive dynamisms lead to integration with resolution or reduction in tension. Sullivan (1953) considers anxiety the chief disruptive force in interpersonal relations and the main factor in the development of serious difficulties in living.

Of importance in the understanding of Sullivan's approach is the strong observational source of knowledge in understanding adult behavior. The development through early childhood is approached largely through inference and hypothesized common experiences. Sullivan describes his formulations as drawing not only from psychoanalytic theory, but from aspects of psychobiology as conceptualized by Meyer and the social psychology of Mead as well as cultural anthropology.

Sullivan defines *man* through what he called the one genus postulate; that man is much more human than otherwise. Born an animal, man develops from this characterization as animal in infancy to a universally determined human personality. Differences between individuals are largely the result of differences in relative maturity of the persons involved. Differences in language and custom also contribute to individuality (Sullivan 1953).

Sullivan listed three principles borrowed from biology[3] that he indicated were a part of his theory. These are communal existence, functional activity, and organization. Communal existence refers to the inseparable nature of the living and the necessary environment with which constant interchange takes place. This constant exchange, through bordering membranes, with the physiochemical universe surrounding him, is essential to man's survival.

All organisms live in continual communal existence, and in constant exchange with the necessary components of their environment. For man, this *environment* necessarily includes culture. The principle of organization includes not only the structure of the organism but the variability of this structure both in the individual and in the race. The principle of functional activity is seen in the interaction of the organism and environment (including component parts of the organism and their environment), or the physiological activity of life (Sullivan 1953).

Health is not specifically addressed. However, the implied definition includes not only the absence of "illness" as inherent in the medical model, but also the predominance of the syntaxic mode of experience. This includes the ability to manage anxiety in such a manner as to promote growth toward maturity (conjunctive dynamism), or to be relatively free of anxiety produced interferences which distort communication (dysjunctive dynamism). Heuristic stages in development as proposed by Sullivan are included in Table 1.

Psychosocial Theory of Erikson

Erik Erikson (1950), beginning as a psychoanalyst, pursued the teachings of Freud, and included the changing perspectives of a new generation of scientists. He offers his interpretations not as a departure from psychoanalysis, but as an elaboration, recognizing the changes he offers as his own experiences and observations of his own time. Moving from the psychosexual to the psychosocial, Erikson added to the trust-mistrust dimension of the oral-sensory stage of development the origin of hope, emanating from a favorable ratio of trust versus mistrust.

In elaborating the anal stage of mastery, Erikson focused not only on mastery of sphincter control, but on the development of the musculature necessary to "will" activity. Thus the crises of this period include

[3] Eldridge S: The Organization of Life, New York, Thomas Y. Crowell Company, 1925

the struggle to go beyond the dependence of "trusting" the mothering one. Again, the resolution of autonomy versus shame and doubt comes not through acceptance of one side of the polarity, but through a favorable ratio toward autonomy; the development of the rudiments of will power. Following this pattern, the rudiments of purpose emerge with the appropriate ratio of initiative versus guilt, competence out of industry versus inferiority, and fidelity out of the identity-role confusion crisis (Table 1). In all of these dimensions, Erikson is suggesting capacity, not specific ideology, and an expectation that the development of these characteristics of maturity will be influenced by the individual capacity and social context within which they develop (Erikson 1964).

He offers as basic principles (1) that one can study the human mind only by engaging the fully motivated partnership of the observed individual and by entering into a sincere contract together; (2) that you will not see in another what you have not learned to recognize in yourself; and (3) that psychological discovery is accompanied by some irrational involvement of the observer, and that it cannot be communicated to another without a certain irrational involvement of both (transference).

His position on women differs markedly from that of Freud. He suggests that Freud's judgment of the identity of women was the weakest part of his theory (Evans 1967), and that it may well have been influenced by the Victorian and patriarchal as well as the sexual mores of his day.

Summary

The psychiatric theories of Freud, Sullivan, and Erikson have been presented in some detail, not only because of their impact on past and current practices in psychiatric mental health nursing, but because of the impact of each on the discipline of nursing. Although psychoanalytic theory as a treatment modality has lost favor in recent years, the remaining impact of component theories on educational and social institutions is widespread. Additionally, it is the basic theory from which most others are described as differing, a tribute, albeit somewhat negative, to its scope.

The impact of Sullivan's interpersonal theory on nursing will be explored more fully as it relates to Peplau's interpersonal model of nursing. Erikson is widely known among those concerned with developmental and life span theories, and has received prominence within nursing generally. However, the derivation of Sullivan's and Erikson's theories from psychoanalysis is often unrecognized. Table 1 reflects a synoptical comparison of these three theories relative to life span development. Primary sources for this information are Freud (1960), Erikson, (1950, 1964), and Sullivan (1953). Additional material may be found in Alexander (1948, 1961), Bellak (1973), and Evans (1967).

Table 1—LIFE SPAN DEVELOPMENT: A COMPARATIVE VIEW

Freud (Psychoanalysis) Biologically based-maturation of nervous system important indicator of libido site, psychosexual development, transformation of energy.		*Sullivan* (Interpersonal Theory)—Relates interpersonal experiences and task mastery. Heuristic stages in development.		*Erikson* (Eight Stages of Man)—Broadens the psychoanalytic base with additional psychosocial input, within concepts of relativity and complementarity.	
Age	*Stage*	*Age*	*Stage*	*Age*	*Stage*
0–1	Oral	0–3	Infancy (Birth to period of articulate speech; differentiation of self)	0–1	Oral–Sensory Stage: *Trust vs. Mistrust*—A balance of the capacity to trust and mistrust in favor of trusting, a sense of being able to get (from mother), and being able to give (satisfaction to mother)
2–3	Anal	3–5	Childhood (Self-system, parallel play)	2–3	Muscular–Anal Stage: *Autonomy vs. Shame and Doubt*—Shame-rage turned against self. A sense of bodily control and self management. A capacity to affect his parents and be affected by them—Language skills develop.
3–6	Phallic (Oedipal)	6–9	Juvenile Era (Associates with companions, learns competition—cooperation, chum period)	4–5	Locomotor–Genital Stage: *Initiative vs. Guilt*—A sense of role in the family. Initiative-anticipatory rivalry.
6–10	Latency	9–12	Preadolescence. Need for interpersonal intimacy with same sex chum.		

12	Genital (Final stage of psychosexual development—begins with puberty and biologic capacity for orgasm) Reproductive Phase	6–11	Latency Stage: *Industry vs. Inferiority*—Social learning (like sharing), precision learning skills (reading math), capacity to work at something.
12	Early Adolescence (Patterning some type of performance to satisfy one's genital drives, begins heterosexual activity)	12–18	Adolescent Stage: *Identity vs. Role Confusion*—A workable identity rather than a sense of self-diffusion, including sexual and social identity. Young Adulthood Stage: *Intimacy vs. Isolation*—Late adolescent to middle age—engage in productive work—share and care about others. Without sharing and caring, you have isolation.
18	Late Adolescence (Patterning of preferred genital activity. Continues to the establishment of fully human or mature repertory of interpersonal relations.) Adulthood: Establishment of love relationship in which other person is nearly as significant as self. Highly developed intimacy with another as major source of satisfaction.		Adulthood Stage: *Generativity vs. Stagnation*—Concerned with others outside immediate family. If generativity isn't developed you stagnate with personal needs and concerns. Old Age & Maturity Stage: *Integrity vs. Despair*—Life needs an end—integrity—individual looks back with satisfaction, despair—too late—missed life's opportunities.
	Phase of Decline — Old Age: Retrogressive changes.		

TREATMENT PERSPECTIVES:

CLINICAL ILLUSTRATION   Throughout this chapter a clinical example will be used to describe the different conceptualizations presented. Recognizing that clinical illustrations must by their very nature be brief, and thus overly simplistic, the example is used to demonstrate the major focus and techniques that differentiate therapeutic approaches. These must be logically consistent with the frameworks from which they are derived.

In this clinical example, an adolescent girl is brought in by her mother for the strangeness of her behavior: "Sometimes she doesn't hear a word I say, and at other times she laughs or cries at the least word!" Sitting off by herself, the girl intently picks at a sore on her hand.

Psychoanalytic Treatment

Man as a biopsychologic organism reacts to his internal and external environment to reduce stress. A major origin of stress, intrapsychic conflict, is managed through mechanisms of defense, learned during the formative years. The health-illness continuum of medical and psychologic models guides interventions toward removal of illness through resolution of unconscious conflicts.

The first major thrust of the intervention in psychoanalysis involves the effort to understand the total dynamic configuration of the personality. Behavioral manifestations are viewed as the natural expressions of fundamental underlying biological dynamics, phylogenetically predetermined, but predetermined to a lesser extent than characteristic of animals. Thus a high degree of molding of the psychodynamic structure of man through later experiences is possible. The study of these molding experiences is recognized as the fundamental contribution of psychoanalysis (Alexander 1961). Further, it is through the recollection and reconstruction of early childhood events, brought into etiological relationship with the present emotional situation which is considered the goal of therapy. Alexander (1961) modifies this therapeutic goal by emphasizing the importance of resolving the transference relationships as a means of recognizing the more intense early relationships that have been repressed.

Addressing the clinical example, the psychoanalytic approach would focus on the adolescent as client. Treatment would begin with an extensive history of the client, and be considered confidential between the girl and her therapist. Since the adolescent is usually able to deal with problems at a verbal level, an attempt would be made to learn from the client the patterns of experience and feelings that would make the dynamic configuration of the personality evident. Through a series of interviews, an attempt would be made to reconstruct the early experiences of childhood to enable the therapist to determine the etiology of the present emotional stress. Uncovering of unconscious conflicts, enabled in part through transference experiences and their resolutions, would be expected.

Sullivan's modifications likely would involve a more active participant observation role by the therapist, and focus more on interaction patterns of interpersonal field. The therapist would seek evidence of the development of conjunctive dynamisms and facilitate this pattern of tension reduction since, within this framework, anxiety is the chief disruptive force in interpersonal relations and the main factor in development of serious problems of living, assessment of anxiety levels, and disjunctive dynamisms. Understanding of conscious and unconscious processes would follow the psychoanalytic model. The adolescent girl in this example probably would be viewed as showing some regression toward experiencing primarily in the parataxic mode, with few experiences in the syntaxic mode. The interpersonal experience with the therapist would be of primary importance, both in diagnosis and treatment. Further explanation can be found in Sullivan (1953) and in the exploration of the Peplau intervention approach, a model drawing heavily on Sullivan's interpersonal theory, but within a nursing perspective.

The treatment approach of *Erikson* is the psychoanalytic model, elaborated with greater emphasis on the social phenomenon. Viewed by Erikson as an extension of psychoanalysis rather than a departure from it, his basic principles emphasize the intrapsychic nature of man, and resolution of transference as a basic component of treatment.

Behavior Modification Framework

Perhaps more specifically called operant conditioning, this framework is derived from the experimental psychology of Watson, enhanced and refined by Skinner. The basic assumptions of this theory include: (1) behavior is learned; (2) behavior occurs in a certain setting or situation; and (3) behavior is maintained or altered by its consequences.

In contrast to theories of intrapsychic and/or interpsychic conflict, the behaviorist has no need of an intervening causative reason or dynamism to account for the behavior. This view is described as a value-free perspective, difficult to achieve, since most people grow up with labels for good and bad, right and wrong behavior. Professional education adds the terms healthy and sick. The behaviorist understands behavior as functional or dysfunctional, adaptive or maladaptive. This is based on an appreciation for the fact that a "person and his behavior are in constant interaction with an external environment" (Loomis and Horsley 1974, p. 4). Certain environmental conditions set the stage for a certain response, followed by certain environmental consequences that influence the future probability of the response.

Behavioral modification is based on an experimental approach wherein the definition of the problem is behaviorally specific. This conceptual framework has evolved inductively out of numerous replications of case studies. It is viewed to be appropriate to the care of any individual who has a problem that can be defined in objective, measurable terms.

Because of the inductive nature of this framework, the more abstract conceptualizations have not been developed. Man is recognized to be more complex than his external behavior alone; however, this framework includes general principles, inductively rather than deductively determined, deriving from extensive replication. Through the control and precise measurement of both dependent and independent variables, this research-based theory continually builds on itself (Loomis et al. 1974).

The Treatment Process

Presented more accurately as a learning process, this approach involves a behavioral assessment followed by a step-by-step process of goal setting and planned behavioral change. Basic to this process is an understanding of the concepts of *operant behavior*, that behavior which operates on the environment to produce a change in that environment. Operant behavior is regulated by its consequences. *Operant responses* are individual units of operant behavior that can be objectively defined and objectively measured, usually in relation to frequency, duration, and/or intensity. *Operant conditioning* consists of the arrangement of responses and stimuli that occur and are strengthened or weakened. *Respondent behavior*, on the other hand, is thought to be governed by its immediate antecedent behavior, thus is elicited by the stimuli. These respondent behaviors, governed by the autonomic nervous system, are described as those behaviors with which an individual is born, and that provide the mechanisms for protection and survival. *Learning* (conditioning) occurs when a new or neutral stimulus that already elicits a response is reinforced. *Reinforcement*, or reinforcing stimuli, affect only the responses immediately preceding them. Positive reinforcement may be achieved either through the provision of a desirable consequence, or the removal of an aversive stimulus (Loomis et al. 1974).

In the clinical example of the young adolescent girl, goals would be behaviorally specific and mutually set, if possible. The regimen would be carefully structured after a determination of the target behavior to be modified, and its frequency, duration, and magnitude. Necessary to this goal setting would be knowledge of who are the primary reinforcers or punishers for this patient, what they do to control the patient's behavior, and what the patient does to control theirs. Additionally, knowledge of the complex chains of behavior performed by the patient, and the conditions currently present in the girl's living and school environments would be needed. To place this approach within the context of an existing nursing conceptual framework, the Roy adaptation model seems most congruent.

COMMUNICATIONS THEORY AND
THEORY OF LOGICAL TYPES
Derived from basic psychoanalytic formulation of the psychic structure wherein ego function is defined precisely as "the process of discriminating communicational modes either within the self or between the self and others," a theory of schizophrenia was proposed by Bateson et al. (1956). An interdisciplinary group, these investigators used a part of communication theory attributed to Russell and called the Theory of Logical Types. The central thesis, that there is discontinuity between a class and its members, is continually and inevitably breached in the psychology of real communication. To elaborate, the class cannot be a member of itself, nor can one of the members be the class, since the term used for class is of a different level of abstraction or a different "Logical Type" than the terms used for its members. This discontinuity characterizes the communication of those persons experiencing schizophrenia (Bateson et al. 1956, 1978).

Assuming that the ego is functionally weak, the schizophrenic demonstrates this weakness in three areas of such functions: (1) difficulty assigning the correct communicational mode to the messages he receives from other persons; (2) difficulty assigning the correct communicational mode to personal verbalizations; and (3) difficult assigning the correct communicational mode to one's own thoughts, sensations, and percepts. Combining learning theory with the evident fact that humans use *context* as a guide for mode discrimination, the schizophrenic's messages to self and others are deviant in syllogistic structure. Rather, the schizophrenic uses structures that identify predicates. He uses unlabeled metaphors. This distortion in communication was thought to result from family interactions in which the sequence of experiences leads to the "double bind."

The *double bind* situation has as its necessary ingredients: (1) two or more persons, one of whom becomes the victim; (2) repeated experiences; (3) a primary negative injunction, usually within the context of learning to avoid punishment; (4) a secondary injunction conflicting with the first at a more abstract level, and like the first, enforced by punishments or signals which threaten survival; and (5) a tertiary negative injunction prohibiting the victim from escaping. Once the individual has learned to perceive his universe in double bind patterns, a no-win situation, almost any portion of the sequence is sufficient to initiate the double bind (Bateson et al. 1956, 1978). This double bind sequence was postulated to produce a breakdown in an individual's ability to discriminate between Logical Types. Thus, this theory proposes family interaction rather than early traumatic experiences as the basis of this symptomatology. To confuse the literal and metaphoric in their own communication when caught in a double bind is also characteristic. The metacommunicative system has broken down. The person is unable to communicate about his communication, that is, the context within which it is to be understood.

An example of the resulting impossible dilemma follows: "If I am to keep my tie to my mother, I must not show her that I love her, but if I do not show her that I love her, I will lose her" (Bateson et al. 1978, p. 19).

Placing this theoretical context in a broader view, Weakland (1978) relates three levels of explanatory schema and their resulting implications for intervention. On the first level, impersonal causation, human events are viewed as consequences of large and powerful external forces. On the second level, personal causation, or problems viewed essentially as consequences of inherent personal characteristics may be causing the immediate problem. The third level, the interactional view, relates what is occurring to interaction within some system of ongoing relationships. This view moves from a linear causal model to a systems approach. Inherent in this is the belief that all parts of the system are interconnected, and all must be studied in the context of the whole. As a consequence of placing their theory within the broader context, these authors have gone beyond the double bind theory to a systems approach.

Further explication of this systems approach to communication is found in Watzlawick et al. (1967). These authors present five tentative axioms as a foundation for this theoretical framework:

1. All behavior in an interactional situation has message value, therefore it is impossible to "not communicate."
2. Every communication has a content and a relationship aspect such that the latter classifies the former and is therefore a metacommunication.
3. The nature of a relationship is contingent upon the punctuation of the communicational sequences between communicants.
4. Human beings communicate both digitally and analogically. Digital language has a highly complex and powerful logical syntax but lacks adequate semantics in the field of relationship, while analogic language possesses the semantics but has no syntax for the unambiguous definition for the nature of relationships.

5. All communicational interchanges are either symmetrical or complementary, depending on whether they are based on equality or difference (Watzlawick et al. 1967).

This communication theory has been widely used in the psychiatric mental health context, especially by those therapists involved in family therapy. The congruence of the theory with King's nursing conceptual framework will be explored.

Maslow's Humanistic Psychology

From his earliest publications in comparative psychology in 1932, until his death in 1970, Abraham Maslow shared his scientific pursuit of the understanding of human behavior. Perhaps best known within the discipline of nursing for his development of a hierarchy of basic needs (Maslow 1954, 1970), Maslow introduced an organized approach to understanding the relationship of biologic and psychologic needs within a total human context.

In the description of *man* as characterized by a hierarchy of basic needs, offered in their order of prepotency, Maslow indicated that need satisfaction leads to the emergence of higher level needs, while need frustration leads to pathology. Beginning with a basic level of need, the physiologic need will be experienced most prominently when all needs are unsatisfied. However, as physiologic needs are satisfied, a higher level of need, categorized by Maslow as safety needs, emerges. Gratification of safety needs might be summarized as the provision of a physical and psychological environment which is familiar, structurally sound, adequately furnished, properly maintained, and conducive to healthy interaction. With relative gratification of safety needs, belonging and love needs emerge. The individual hungers for affectionate relationships, a sense of belonging, a place within his group. Maslow attributed frustration of these needs as the most commonly found core in maladjustment and psychopathology. With gratification of these needs emerges the esteem needs, for self respect or self esteem and for the esteem of others, basic to the continued emergence of identity and development of potential toward adequacy, social conscience, and purpose.

The unidirectional nature of man evolving is clear within this hierarchy, for relative gratification of the esteem needs leads to the emergence of need for self actualization. This is described as the desire to become more and more what one is capable of becoming (Maslow 1954). This emphasis on self actualization is congruent with and widely accepted in nursing.

As he continued to test empirically these hypotheses, Maslow indicated: ". . . basic human needs can be fulfilled *only* by and through other human beings, i.e., society. The need for community (belongingness, contact, groupness) is itself a basic need. Loneliness, isolation, ostracism, rejection by the group—these are not only painful but pathogenic as well . . . humaness and specieshood in the infant is only a potentiality and must be actualized by the society" (Maslow 1971, p. 347).

In this later work, Maslow is clearly reaching beyond a particulate view toward a more and more inclusive view of man's nature. In studying self-actualizing individuals, he developed a theory of metamotivation. Self-actualizing persons are gratified in all of their basic needs and thus are no longer motivated by them, yet in some, higher needs emerge and create what he calls metamotivation (Maslow 1971).

In addressing the topic "Toward a Humanistic Biology," Maslow (1971) presents the concern that psychology is being torn into three or more separate non-communicating sciences or groups of scientists. The first group he identifies as comprising the behavioristic, objectivistic, mechanistic, positivistic groups. The second group comprises all those psychologies that originated in Freud and in psychoanalysis. The third group, described as the humanistic psychologies, and often thought to be the "third force," is a coalescense of various splinter groups into a single philosophy. Although he acknowledges that many within this third group see themselves as opposed to one or both of the previous groups, Maslow believes the third psychology to include the first two. To interpret this, he comes to the terms "epi-Freudian" and "epi-behavioristic" to indicate that each are built upon (epi = upon) the others.

Maslow has further stated a desire to develop a psychology of transcendence. Suggesting that a value-free, value-neutral, and value-avoiding model of science is unsuitable for the study of life, he proposes a research design based upon the selection, not of a random sample, but of a superior sample from which to study the questions of greatest importance in regard to the development of the human potential. To deal with this research design, he proposes the development of "growing tip statistics," a title taken from the fact that the greatest genetic action in plants takes place at the tip (Maslow 1971, p. 7).

Maslow further declared that human history comprises a record of the ways in which human nature has been sold short. He stated that the highest possibilities of human nature have practically always been underrated. Maslow cites evidence to support the humanistic-psychological point of view, that the data are on the side of self regulation, self government, and self choice of the organism. Implications of these findings on the image of the scientist, no matter in what field, are indicative of a shift from a controlling to a more Taoistic image. Taoistic is used by Maslow to summarize non-intruding, non-controlling. It means asking rather than controlling, and stresses non-interfering observation rather than a controlling manipulation. In his view, the "good psychotherapist" is of this Taoist image. So, too, is the parent, teacher, lover, and friend, cast in the Taoist image as most supportive of human growth and self-actualization (Maslow 1971).

The concept of *environment*, in Maslow's model, is implicit rather than explicit. Providing both means for gratification and frustration, the social context is a highly potent factor in human development.

The man-environment interaction is explicit: "not only is man *part* of nature, and it a part of him, but also he must be at least isomorphic with nature (similar to it) in order to be viable in it. It has evolved him. His communion with what transcends him therefore need not be defined as non-natural or super-natural. It may be seen as a biological experience" (Maslow 1971, p. 332).

Biological is elaborated by Maslow to be synonymous with, or to include evolutionary emergence. Maslow's commitment to a concept of *health*, which goes beyond the usual definition of absence of illness, is well elaborated in the concept of self-actualization. Although he speaks of a health-illness continuum, he more frequently indicates an emergence of full humaness as goal, and of deprivation as leading to diminution of humaness. In developing a theory of "metamotivation" he indicates the emergence of "metaneeds" which include the "highest" values, the spiritual life, and the highest aspirations of mankind (Maslow 1971).

The approach to the hypothetical client will be explored through The Unitary Man Model of Nursing Science proposed by Rogers, with which this theory is most congruent.

NURSING MODELS:
PEPLAU'S INTERPERSONAL
MODEL OF NURSING In defining the correlate, *person*, Peplau emphasizes the perspective of human needs, that when unmet, lead to demands for satisfaction. The management of the tension experienced from unmet needs is a major factor in the shaping of behavior. She describes man's behavior as purposeful and goal seeking in terms of feelings of satisfaction and/or security. Further, any interference with, blocking of, or barrier to, a need, drive, or desired goal before satisfaction of these urges has been achieved constitutes frustration. Frustrations are further related to the levels of aspirations that individuals set for themselves (Peplau 1952).

Environment, or social context, is discussed in two major ways. The nurse, as a part of the patient's environment or social context, has a major impact on the individual's response. Environment, generally, is described as including conditions essential for experiencing health.

These conditions, although not fully understood, are believed to include both physical demands and interpersonal conditions. The physical demands of the human organism require material conditions manipulated in behalf of the welfare of an individual or group. Interpersonal conditions that are both individual and social, meet personality needs and allow the expression and use of capacities in a productive way.

Health is described by Peplau as "a word symbol that implies forward movement of personality and other ongoing human processes in the direction of creative, constructive, productive, personal, and community living" (1952, p. 12). Additionally, nurses participate with other professional workers in the organization of conditions that facilitate the forward movement toward health. Nurses share in the responsibility for the development of criteria for "desirable living," and for working out plans and policies for achieving development of conditions that make health possible (Peplau 1952).

"*Nursing*, like other professions, is primarily an applied science. It uses established knowledge for beneficial purposes" (Peplau 1969, p. 33). From this perspective, it would seem that the direct acceptance of useable concepts from other disciplines is appropriate. The key to development of a theory-based nursing practice is in the process of selection of concepts to the purpose at hand. However, as she further develops her conceptualization of theory in nursing, Peplau moves beyond this approach.

First she differentiates concepts from processes, the latter being an organization of concepts into larger components or phases, occurring in serial order and showing the emergence of particular behaviors (i.e., the developmental process). Peplau believes that concepts generally derive from empirical observations, and that "nursing situations provide a field of observations from which unique nursing concepts can be derived and used for the improvement of the professional's work" (p. 36). This then implies the beginnings of a science of nursing. The unique focus of nursing rests in the reactions of the patient or client to the circumstances of his illness or health problem. This focus was elaborated by Dorothy Gregg and cited by Peplau as "helping patients to gain intellectual and interpersonal competencies beyond that which they have at the point of illness . . ." (Peplau 1969, p. 37). The overlapping with medicine occurs only when dealing with the disease processes more directly.

Nursing is further elaborated by Peplau as a process through which nurses may assume any of six identified roles. An initial role, that of *stranger*, includes the sharing of respect and positive interest in the client. In the stranger role, the nurse is at first nonpersonal; offers the same ordinary courtesies that are accorded a guest brought into any new situation. This implies accepting the patient as he or she is, and relating to the patient as an emotionally able stranger until or unless evidence shows him or her to be otherwise.

A second role, that of *resource person*, provides specific answers to questions usually formulated to address a larger problem. The third role, *teacher*, includes combinations of all other roles. The *leadership* role relates to activities toward development of democratic leadership, even within clinical situations. The role of *surrogate* arises in situations where there is need for resolution within the interpersonal process. Surrogate roles are determined by psychological age factors operating by reasons of arrests in development, feelings reactivated through the experience of illness or on the basis of demands made by individuals in a clinical situation. A nurse helps the patient to learn that there are likenesses and differences between people, and by being herself assists with the needed resolution.

The role of *counselor* provides for the meeting of the major purpose of all nurse-patient relationships, that of promoting experiences leading to health. This is accomplished through a series of immediate goals. Helping a patient become aware of conditions required for health, providing these conditions when possible, identifying threats to health, and using the evolving interpersonal events to facilitate learning are the steps toward achievement of this purpose (Pelau 1952).

Intervention

Since nursing is viewed by Peplau as an interpersonal process (Peplau 1952, 1969), intervention begins with the development of a relationship with the patient. Phases of the nurse-patient relationship outlined within this model, and widely accepted throughout nursing practice, include orientation, identification, exploitation, and resolution. Although described as distinct phases, overlapping is expected throughout the relationship. The roles or functions common to nursing practice that were described previously are interlocking, and may be seen in any combination during the phases of the relationship. An important aspect of the relationship in orientation (phase 1) is in helping patients become aware of the availability of these roles and functions as they are needed by the patient.

Phase two, identification, is enhanced when the nurse permits the patients to express what they feel and still receive all of the nursing care they need. This permits the experiencing of illness as an opportunity to re-orient feelings and strengthen the positive forces of the personality. Patients tend to respond to this experience in one of three ways, as a independent participant in the relationship with a nurse, as an independent in isolation from the nurse, or as a dependent participant displaying helplessness and dependence upon the nurse.

Phase three, exploitation, represents the major working phase, wherein the patient derives full value from the relationship in accordance with his view of the situation. The final phase, resolution, refers not so much to the problems engaged during the working phase, but to the gradual freeing from identification with the helping professional and the generation and strengthening of the ability to stand more or less alone.

Following the Peplau model with the adolescent girl, the orientation phase of the relationship would provide the opportunity for the client to experience the respect, positive interest, and expectation for appropriate response. The orientation to available resources, including roles and functions of the nurse, provides a base for exploring new ways of coping with anxiety, and opportunities for expression of feelings in a non-punitive relationship. Problems of identification within the relationship, like transference relationships in psychoanalysis, offer a new opportunity to modify patterns of relating through re-experiencing early conflictual situations with different outcomes. One would expect particular attention to development of an independent participant relationship with the nurse as the working phase (exploitation) evolves in the relationship, to avoid the increased retreat and regression likely in this troubled young client. Resolution of this relationship would focus on the emancipation of the adolescent for continued self-directed activities designed to manage tension successfully, permitting the emergence of more mature needs.[4]

OREM SELF CARE
MODEL   Man is viewed as an integrated whole, a unity functioning biologically, symbolically, and socially. The societal influence is strong in the Orem model, and reflected in the man-environment interaction. She speaks of needed environmental conditions as either physical or social, and refers to the socializing process as significant. She further discusses internally oriented behaviors necessary in self-care as those dependent upon awareness, perception, and decision making as related to self and environment, and upon a state of motivation and interest necessary to learning and applying knowledge. Emotions are only mentioned as something in need of control in order to face the reality of one's health situation.

Orem presents man and environment as an integrated system related to self care, with human functioning highly integrated at every stage of the life cycle. Understanding of this aspect of human-

---

[4] For the psychiatric nurse therapist, specific techniques and strategies of Peplau's investigative approach to psychotherapy may be found in Field, WE, The Psychotherapy of Hildegard Peplau. New Brounfels, Texas, PSF Productions, 1979.

environmental interaction requires knowledge of anatomic structure, physiologic mechanisms, and unique patterns for responding to environmental stimuli. Implications for both universal and relative perspectives are inherent in this approach. Further, Orem indicates that man's functioning, linked to environment as an integrated functional whole or system, can be altered safely only within narrow limits. Thus, universality is recognized as predominant.

Adaptive forces, both within man's nature and within the environment, as well as creative forces of individual members of social groups, contribute toward the development of techniques used by persons to control themselves, their environment, and their dependents. Concepts such as adaptation, along with implicit causation, and the expectation that deliberative effort to introduce new elements into the environment may effect the balance of the system, are indicative of a somewhat, or sometimes, closed system. The concept of holism within this model is additive.

Orem defines *health* as "state of wholeness or integrity of the individual human being, his parts, and his modes of functioning" (Orem 1971, p. 42). She broadens this definition, stating that it "implies the capacity to live as a human being within one's physical, biologic, and social environment, achieving some measure of the human life potential as distinguished from the potential of other forms of life." Health is the responsibility of a total society and all of its members, involving many "health roles." Because the definition of health is to some extent dependent upon one's views of man's human and biologic characteristics, and the philosophic view related to a given discipline is emphasized, various definitions will emerge. The health-illness continuum is implied with universal self-care and health-deviation self-care defining the ends of the continuum.

According to Orem (1971) *nursing* is a human service, arising out of a mandate from society. Like other human services, nursing is a way of overcoming human limitations. It is a personal, family, and community service within the health field, but focuses primarily on the individual, regardless of the context. "Nursing has as its special concern man's need for self-care action and the provision and management of it on a continuous basis in order to sustain life and health, recover from disease or injury, and cope with their effects" (Orem 1971).

Nursing care as viewed by Orem may be continuous or periodic, and has both health and illness dimensions. The two main conceptual elements of nursing are (1) self-care, including universal self-care and health deviation self-care, and (2) self-care inabilities or limitations. The formal object of nursing rests with the inabilities of individuals to engage in self-care because of health or health related reasons. The results are specified in relation to self-care and self-care agency. The boundaries defined for nursing include: (1) may be required by any age group, but the situation of health, not the dependencies arising from age, initiate the requirements for nursing; (2) the requirements for nursing may be modified by progressive favorable change in the state of health of the individual or increased learning or capacity to be self-directing in self-care. Nursing's relationships in society are based on a state of imbalance between the abilities of nurses to manage and maintain systems of therapeutic self-care for individuals and the abilities of the individuals and their families to do this. When nurses' abilities are greater there is a valid need for service; if equal, or individual or family's ability is greater there is no valid basis for service.

The concepts of man, nursing, and health as described by Orem are interwoven. The major unifying force seems to be society which defines *health*, mandates agency (at times the responsibility of the adult in the society and at times the responsibility of nursing or medicine), spells out clearly under what conditions the agency may belong to the nurse, under what conditions patiency (receiver of service) is acceptable, and the credentials for, and the scope of, the practice of nursing. The broad system—society—thus has a major influence over the man-environment system and the particular nursing system selected for the situation (see Figure 1).

Through the nursing process, the nurse selects the nursing model appropriate to the patient, designs more specifically the system including the nursing situations (helping situations in which patient requirements for care and abilities and assisting acts of the nurse bring about a complementary set of behaviors). The core element of the nursing situation includes what the nurse and patient must do to achieve health goals for the patient. The person elements include the patient as a person with all of the contributions of age, sex, physical, intellectual, and emotional manifestations of growth and development, characteristic behaviors, cultural manifestations, past and present external demands. The nurse is seen as a person with position factors, role as agent, acceptance of, and willingness to render, care. The core elements and person elements combined with the health and disease elements comprise the total. Figure 2 is a schematic representation of these relationships.

The Orem Self Care Model of nursing has many points congruent with those of Peplau. Additionally, Orem's model is congruent in several aspects with psychoanalysis, but is more congruent with Sullivan. Perhaps the best fit is with Erikson's modified and expanded view of the psychoanalytic perspective, which provides the social context required for the Orem model. Additionally, through the developmental approach, the healthy conflict resolution at each stage, leading to the

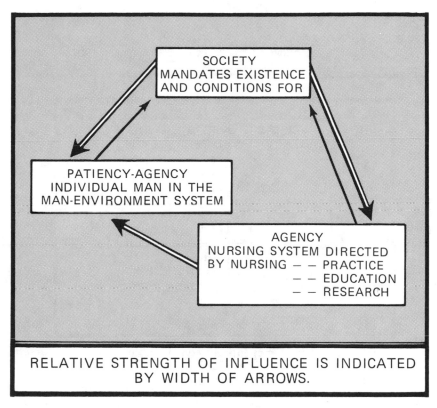

Figure 1.—Orem Self Care Model: Interrelationships Among Concepts.

virtues of hope, will power, competence, fidelity, etc., as a basic under-standing are congruent with the developing capacity for self-care agency of the Orem model.

Elaboration and extension of the nature of man to a holistic system are necessary in the reformulation of the Eriksonian approach within the Orem framework. Although Erikson attends to aspects of the bio-psychosocial nature of man, the emphasis is still largely intrapsychic. Orem recognizes the system within which the individual functions, more fully explores the agency role shared between client and therapist, and, in the example used, would perhaps involve the mother more fully in the shared agency function, since the adolescent is not expected to assume full self-care agency. Assessment of self-care capacity of both the girl and her mother would lead to selection of the nursing system most suited to the intervention. Whether the supportive-educative or the partially compensatory system would be best suited would depend on the determined relationship between self-care capacities, or self-

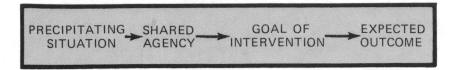

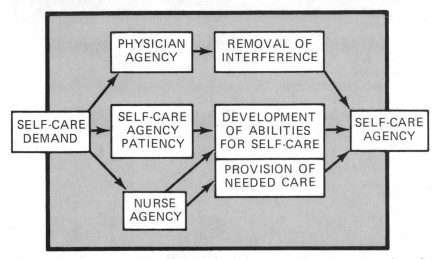

Figure 2.—Roles in Therapeutic Intervention Reflecting Interdisciplinary Approach (Orem Self-Care Model).

care deficit and self-care demand. Recommendations for hospitalization versus outpatient treatment would depend, to a large extent, on the balance of socially mandated and inappropriate behaviors.

THE BEHAVIORIST VIEW

OF NURSING   Loomis and Horsley have already reformulated behavior modification for use within the discipline of nursing to the extent that they place it within a broader context. Stating that nurses need a theoretical framework that will help them view the whole person within the context of his environment, these authors indicate that nursing is the only discipline with the "time and ability to regard the patient as a total physical, emotional, and social being . . . their sphere of expertise should be in the area of assisting patients to modify their maladaptive personal and interpersonal behaviors so that they can assume a more adaptive position in society" (1974, p. 9).

Nursing is a practice-oriented profession involved with the behavior of people who need help. According to the behaviorist view, nurses need a psychology that: (1) is based on a purpose similar to that of the patient-care situation; (2) uses terminology appropriate for classifying events in the area of practice; (3) includes concepts broadly applicable to numerous patient-care problems and practice situations; (4) has an inclusive approach to the individual and his interaction with his environment; (5) contains manipulative variables that the nurse can use in assessing patient problems. These authors believe that nursing has suffered in the twentieth century from the progress of the nineteenth, in which maladaptive behavior was viewed as "mental illness." This medical model often gets in the way of making patients and their supporting environments responsible participants in the treatment process. It has influenced nursing care delivery through the illness theory and the reliance on treating the underlying cause of the presenting symptom. The implication of this approach, that a behavior disorder cannot be approached directly, relies on the expectation of some underlying conflict or disturbance to be removed (Loomis et al. 1974).

THE ROY ADAPTATION
MODEL
Like Orem and King, Roy views the holistic nature of man from an additive perspective. *Man* is a biopsychosocial being. The person contains a biologic component, including anatomy and physiology, as well as psychologic and social components. Behavior of the person is related to behavior of others on a group level. Roy states that the "methods of analysis of the person must come from the biologic, psychologic, and social sciences and the person as a unified whole must be viewed from these perspectives" (Roy 1980, p. 180). The person as a biopsychosocial being is in constant interaction with a changing environment, confronting constant physical, social, and psychologic changes in his environment. He learns or acquires mechanisms from each of these spheres that are used to cope with the environmental changes impinging upon him. Responding positively to these changes requires adaptation, and brings about health. Illness, or maladaptation, occurs when the stimuli impinging upon the person are outside the adaptive zone, that is, beyond the level or range of stimuli to which the individual can respond positively.

The person is characterized by two primary adaptive mechanisms, the cognator and regulator, either of which may be utilized in any of the four adaptive modes—physiologic, self concept, role function and interdependence relations. The adaptive zone is the range of stimuli that can be accommodated positively by the individual through his primary mechanisms in any or all of his adaptive modes. Stimuli that must be accommodated include three levels—focal, contextual, or residual. It is in the area of these stimuli and the extent to which they may be manipulated and modified that nursing interventions are expected to focus.

Nursing's goal is the person's adaptation in all of his or her four adaptive modes. The nursing action is the action used to change the course of events toward the desired patient adaptation. Thus, the nurse acts as an external regulatory force to modify stimuli affecting adaptation. The nurse's mode of intervention is to increase, decrease, or maintain stimulation. This takes place within the nursing process (Roy 1980).

Reformulating Behaviorism Within the Roy Adaptation Model

Although there is considerable congruence in intervention modalities, the Roy model has explicated the holistic nature of man and includes a more extensive process of assessment. The behavioral inventory described for behavior modification provides for needed assessment of the focal stimuli leading to maladaptive behavior. This approach utilizes both the strengthening of adaptive behaviors and decreasing the strength of maladaptive behaviors. Roy focuses on modification of the stimuli without addressing expected or nonexpected modifications in the adaptive modes (see Figure 3).

KING SYSTEMS

MODEL   King views nursing as a system, functioning as a part of many social systems, changed by and altering itself in response to changing social forces within a culture. For King, reciprocal impact that nursing may have on the society and its institutions seems more viable. The systems within which nurses work, according to the King model, are designated by the focus within the social system, i.e., personal systems focusing on individuals, interpersonal systems focusing on groups, and the social systems focusing on the wider society. Basic concepts inherent within each of these include: perceptions, information, and energy within the personal system; interpersonal relations and communications within the interpersonal system; and social organization and role status within the society at large (King 1971).

King indicates that the framework for nursing is social systems. The methods of nursing are largely interpersonal relationships determined by perception and health. Perception is defined as each individual's representation or image of reality. She cautions that it is imperative for nurses to be aware of the disparity that often exists between behaviors from which concepts are identified, and the meaning of behavior and concept to the individuals involved.

Nursing is a process of action, reaction, interaction, and transaction whereby nurses assist individuals of any age and socioeconomic group to meet their basic needs in performing activities of daily living and to cope with health and illness at some particular point in the life cycle.

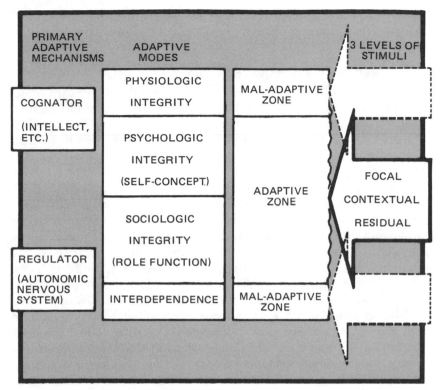

Figure 3.—Roy Adaptation Model. This model has been reformulated to include, as alternative strategies for intervention, efforts to increase the range of the adaptive zone. This is accomplished through increased development or modification of any of the four adaptive modes, as well as through altering stimuli.

Man is a reacting, time-oriented, social being who functions in social systems through interpersonal relationships. Perception of objects, persons, and events influences relationships, and thus life and health.

Health is a dynamic state in the life cycle of man attained through continuous adaptation to stress in the internal and external environments. Through optimum use of resources, maximum potential for growth, development, and for daily living are achieved.

Environment is not explicitly defined in this model. However, King refers to the model as a systems approach and indicates that there is interaction between the internal and external environments of man. Further, she indicates that the nursing situation is the immediate environment, the spatial and temporal reality within which the nurse and client establish a relationship. With concepts of action, reaction, and interaction, the man-environment system implicitly moves from closed to open. For King, the concept of holism is an additive approach.

CONGRUENCE OF KING SYSTEMS MODEL
WITH COMMUNICATION THEORY
An additive or summative approach to holism as implied in the King model is incongruent with Watzlawick's presentation. He cites nonsummativity as a corollary of the notion of wholeness. Further, Watzlawick contrasts individual-oriented approaches with communication theory and indicates that communication sequences would be reciprocally inseparable, in short, that interaction is nonsummative (Watzlawick et al. 1967, p. 126). Within the discussion of the nursing process, the action-reaction portion of the process (King) may be perceived as inconsistent with the interaction-transaction component. The former seems to relate more specifically with a closed system interpretation, or a unilateral, causal approach; the latter more clearly an open systems complimentarity. Similar criticism has been leveled at the communications theorists who also maintain closed systems concepts within their interaction model. The major thrust of the King model is interpreted here as congruent with the communication theory presented. Both the communications theoretical framework and the King systems model direct intervention toward the ongoing interaction process of the client and significant others. Presenting appraisal of the adolescent girl by the mother might well lead to the exploration of interaction patterns for additional evidence of disconfirmation of the girl by her mother, and perhaps others, in communication, and a repeated pattern of "double bind" or paradoxical communication as precipitating the present symptoms.

ROGERS' UNITARY MAN
MODEL
The science of *unitary man* conceptualizes man as a four-dimensional energy field in mutual interaction with *environment*, a four-dimensional energy field, changing together over time. The nature of the change, nonlinear unidirectionality, is toward increasing diversity and complexity of pattern and organization. The concept of unidirectionality within the context of open systems implies a continuous negentropic developmental process. Thus, the holistic person is a four-dimensional, negentropic energy field identified by pattern and organization and manifesting characteristics and behaviors that are different from those of the parts, and that cannot be predicted from knowledge of those parts (Rogers 1980).

The assumptions on which this model is based emphasize the

openness of the man-environment system. Differing from the previously discussed models in degree of consistency with open systems concepts and the rejection of closed systems concepts, concepts of universality, emergence, and unidirectionality are compatible.

The Rogers' conceptual framework posits the man-environment energy field as coextensive with the universe. The developmental process is characterized by variations in pattern and organization. Identified correlates include temporality, or nonlinear temporal rhythms, movement, consciousness, and perceptual experiences (Fitzpatrick 1980).

Health is viewed by Rogers as symphonic interaction of holistic persons and their environments. *Nursing* is understood first as a noun. Nursing is the science of unitary man. Nursing practice is viewed as the facilitation of symphonic interaction between the holistic person and environment.

IMPLICATIONS FOR NURSING

PRACTICE   Nursing practice, influenced by the medical model, has been characterized by a unified commitment to health care and to holism, a commitment often conflictually coupled with a particulate, linear, causal approach to illness prevention or treatment. Most conceptual frameworks have characterized man's progress through life as an inevitable decline following the reproductive years (Freud 1960, Erikson 1950, Sullivan 1953). Even with the move toward inclusion of systems theory, the closed system concept of entropy has been most widely accepted. Man is variously described as being at the mercy of either his internal or external environment. An important exception to this perspective is found in the work of Maslow previously discussed. His description of the self-actualized person, and the emerging concepts of metaneeds and metamotivation are clearly compatible with Rogers' conceptual framework. Rogers' view however, as an open systems approach, is broader than the psychology proposed by Maslow. Maslow's proposal for a psychology of transcendence was left undeveloped by his sudden death in 1970.

A major implication of Rogers' conceptual framework, man as an open system, innovative, emerging, becoming, is the recognition of ongoing developmental phases, rather than the reaching of a peak or plateau, inevitably followed by a decline. Another point of congruence between Maslow's theoretical framework and the Rogers' model is in the Taoistic approach to therapeutic intervention. Rogers' approach is facilitative, not controlling or invasive.

One might speculate that within the Rogers' framework, the nurse therapist would take a life history of the presenting client within the context of the environmental field. Rhythm profiles for the adolescent and her significant others would be important. Since this theory postulates both ontogenetic and phylogenetic emergence, one would anticipate variation in pattern and organization, encourage tolerance of uniqueness, and facilitate the accomodation of generational as well as developmental differences among the interacting parties. The adolescent's behavior would be viewed within the context of her own pattern and organization, including her pattern of valuing. Alternative patterns would be offered when asynchronous patterns are identified.

Similar assistance would be offered to the mother. Accommodation of differences could be facilitated best when each participant more clearly views his or her own pattern and organization, and perception of the patterns of others. When the nurse therapist's patterns of valuing differ from those of the clients, recognition of these as alternative patterns for consideration, rather than as imposed goals, is important. The valuing patterns of the given society must be recognized in facilitating accommodation of divergent life styles.

SUMMARY   The major psychiatric theories from which many psychiatric-mental health nurses have derived psychotherapeutic interventions were reviewed. Through exploration of the definitions and assumptions about man, environment and health, differences were identified. Explication of differences in treatment approaches by means of a clinical example was offered.

As a step in the development of theory based practice within the discipline of nursing, the major existing nursing models were presented. Congruence-incongruence between psychiatric theories and nursing models was viewed through the use of mechanistic, organismic, and relational paradigms. Using the issues of external versus internal locus of developmental change, reductionism versus emergence, unidirectionality versus bidirectionality and universality versus relativity, positions on these issues were related to the paradigms. Theories and models with the most congruence were then compared and needed reformulations identified. The incompatibility among psychiatric theories and nursing models highlights the need for viewing each borrowed theory within the context of a nursing conceptual framework. Reformulation can then occur, enabling a theory-based practice that is logically consistent, and that gives needed direction to practice and research. From this process, psychiatric mental health nurses can continue to develop and test both theory and intervention strategies that will articulate nursing's contribution both to mental health care recipients and providers.

References

Aldous J: Strategies for developing family theory. J Marriage Family, 32:250–257, 1970

Alexander F: Fundamentals of Psychoanalysis. New York, Norton, 1948

Alexander F: The Scope of Psychoanalysis: Selected Papers of Franz Alexander. New York, Basic Books, 1961

Bateson G, Jackson DD, Haley J, Weakland J: Toward a theory of schizophrenia. Behav Sci, 1:251–264, 1956 Reprinted in Berger M (Ed.) Beyond the Double Bind, New York, Brunner-Mazel, 1978.

Bellak M, Gediman HK: Ego Functions in Schizophrenics, Neurotics, and Normals. New York, John Wiley and Sons, 1973

Eldridge S: The Organization of Life. New York, Thomas T. Crowell Co., 1925

Erikson E: Childhood and Society. New York, Norton, 1950

Erikson E: Insight and Responsibility. New York. Norton, 1964

Evans RI: Dialogue with Erik Erikson. New York, Harper and Row, 1967

Fitzpatrick JJ: Patients' perceptions of time: current research. Int Nurs Rev, 27:148–153, 1980

Freud S: The Ego and the Id. New York, Norton, 1960

Hultsch D, Plemons J: Life events and lifespan development. In Baltis P, Brimm O (Eds.): Life Span Development and Behavior. New York, Academic Press, 1979

King IM: Toward a Theory for Nursing. New York, John Wiley & Sons, 1971

Loomis M, Horsely J: Interpersonal Change: A Behavioral Approach to Nursing Practice. New York, McGraw-Hill, 1974

Maslow AH: Motivation and Personality. New York, Harper & Bros., 1954

Maslow AH: Motivation and Personality (rev. ed.), New York, Harper & Row, 1970

Maslow AH: The Farther Reaches of Human Nature. New York, Viking Press, 1971

Nursing Development Conference Group. Concept formalization in nursing. Boston, Little, Brown & Co., 1973

Orem DE: Nursing: Concepts of Practice. New York, McGraw-Hill, 1971

Peplau H: Interpersonal Relationships in Nursing: A Conceptual Frame of Reference for Psychodynamic Nursing. New York, G. P. Putnam's Sons, 1952

Peplau H: Theory: the professional dimension. In Norris M (Ed.): Proceedings of the First Nursing Theory Conference. University of Kansas Medical Center, Department of Nursing Education, March, 1969

Rogers ME: The Theoretical Basis of Nursing. Philadelphia, F. A. Davis, 1970

Rogers ME: Nursing: A science of unitary man. *In* Reihl J, Roy C (Eds.): Conceptual Models for Nursing Practice (2nd ed.), New York, Appleton-Century-Crofts, 1980

Roy C: The Roy adaptation model. *In* Reihl J, Roy C (Eds.): Conceptual Models for Nursing Practice (2nd ed.), New York, Appleton-Century-Crofts, 1980

Sullivan HS: The Interpersonal Theory of Psychiatry. New York, W. W. Norton & Company, Inc., 1953

Watzlawick P, Beavin JH, Jackson DD: Pragmatics of Human Communication. New York, W. W. Norton, 1967

Weakland J: Pursuing the evident into schizophrenia and beyond. *In* Berger M (Ed.): Beyond the Double Bind, New York, Brunner-Mazel, 1978

4 FAMILY SYSTEM THEORY: RELATIONSHIP TO NURSING CONCEPTUAL MODELS

Ann L. Whall

Kaplan (1963) stated that fields of knowledge know no boundaries, that is, no one discipline "owns" a particular area. All disciplines are therefore free to "borrow" from one another, but just as surely must reformulate that knowledge according to their own discipline. Nursing for the most part has borrowed theories of family functioning as presented within other disciplines without bothering to reformulate (Whall 1980).

This chapter presents the reformulation of one substantive knowledge area, family systems theory, according to what, in a sense, is the syntax of nursing, the nursing models. However, just as the past influences the future, the substantive knowledge base of family theory is patterned by its own past. But before the background of family systems theory is discussed, a few points need to be made.

The approach to family theory used here is to consider as a family systems theory any theory that views family in a unitary manner, and considers the members to be interacting parts of that unit. A second point is that, although family systems theories are related to general systems theories, few theorists discuss the family system using the terminology of a pure systems theorist. Rather, such terms as systems, subsystems, open systems, closed systems, and optimal system state dominate the family systems discussions. Therefore these terms and others are used in this chapter. Finally, there are many ways to classify family systems theories. Some consider group dynamics and communication theories to be forerunners of family systems theory. Although this is undoubtedly true, there are other disciplines and approaches that have had greater influence on the family systems perspective, and that nursing uses more often. These influences are from sociology, from the crisis perspective, and from the psychologically based family therapy theories. These approaches are discussed initially in relation to each other. Certain therapy theories are then analyzed according to the nursing models of Rogers (1970, 1980), Orem (1980), and Roy (1976).

BACKGROUND OF FAMILY
SYSTEMS THEORY   Family systems theory has a rather varied
past. The approach to the family system found in sociology and family
therapy theories, however, are quite distinct. In the early stages of
family theory development, the field was dominated by the family
sociologists. By perusing the early sociological journals, one can identify that theory building efforts, at least in terms of research, have
focused primarily on exploratory and exploratory-descriptive studies. A
good example of an early family system theory building effort from the
discipline of sociology is the work of Hill (1949) in "Families Under
Stress." Considered a forerunner of the crises approach to families, Hill
describes the family as a living system, a group of interrelated persons,
that changes over time acting, reacting, and changing in response to
the challenges of wartime separation, loss, and reunion. In this early
study, Hill did not emphasize the term family systems; this was to come
later.

Nye and Berardos' (1966) work, *Emerging Conceptual Frameworks
in Family Analysis*, identified a great deal of variability in the sociological and other approaches to the study of the family system. The 11 plus
conceptual frameworks that were identified included the major frameworks discussed earlier by Hill, Katz, and Simpson (1957). In rereading
the early conceptual models such as the structural functional and situational approaches, the reader is struck with the diversity that springs
from different approaches when viewing data. In an approach sometimes called the home economics approach, for example, the focus is
on the family-environmental interchange. The family is seen as a system bartering, conserving, and exchanging within the environmental
setting. Conversely, in the structural functional approach, the focus is
definitely on the internal family structure and function, e.g., role structure and the concomitant functional patterns. The importance of the
conceptual model used to view the data becomes most evident when
the same phenomenon, the family system, is examined from the differing perspectives of the various sociological frameworks.

Family sociologists have attempted to classify the family frameworks, but in general, these theoretical positions have changed over
time and some are no longer distinguishable (Broderick 1971, Hill and
Hansen 1960). Hill (1974) discusses the relationship between the
structural-functional and developmental approaches and the modern
family systems model. Influenced by one another, the sociological conceptual frameworks have thus tended to merge, the result has many
times been to approach the family from more of a systems perspective.

An additional component of family systems theory is that developed by the family therapists. Psychologically based and less interested
in exploring and describing primarily "what is" than the sociologists,

the therapists were concerned with what could be done to facilitate change in "dysfunctional" families. The theory developed by the therapists is therefore concerned with what is most functional to the family both in terms of the individual and the group. The first statements of this new family systems approach are found in the early writings of Jackson (1957), Ackerman (1967), Haley (1959) and others. This family systems approach does not have a very long history. Napier and Whitaker (1978) discuss that the therapy theories that viewed the family as a system were very long in developing because the first half of the nineteenth century was dominated by individual therapy approaches.

Although psychiatric mental health nursing has been influenced by both the sociological and family therapy approaches to the family system, by far the greatest influence is that of the family therapists. This influence is perhaps because of differences both in the intent and level of theory. Whereas the sociologists discussed variables to be measured when describing or exploring the family system, the therapists were more concerned with assessing specific family functioning, identifying and treating problem areas. The difference in the theory produced by the two disciplines is more readily understood by the schema developed by Donaldson and Crowley (1978). There are academic disciplines and professional disciplines; within the professional disciplines, questions regarding practice are entertained. The academic discipline seeks to describe and explore in order to understand, not treat. Thus the family systems theory developed by the sociologists is less readily applicable to treatment issues.

A third historical portion of the family systems approach is that of the crisis theorists. Stemming from the early work of Lindemann (1944) and Hill (1949), there was an explication of the crises perspective with regard to the family system. Parad and Caplan (1965) developed a model for family assessment that was related to this crises perspective.

In terms of specificity of treatment, however, the family systems theories developed by therapists are much more specific and detailed than either the sociological or crises approaches. Thus, the family systems theories discussed in the remainder of this chapter are those of the family therapists.

GENERIC FEATURES OF THE FAMILY SYSTEM

APPROACHES   There are several common approaches to the family system utilized by the family therapists. Those discussed here are the unitary conceptualizations of the family system, the assumption of some optimal functional state, be it homeostasis, equilibrium, or synchrony, and the assumption that the system is an open system, a closed system, or some variation of these.

Perhaps the most important feature of the family systems approach is that of a unitary conceptualization of family. By mid-twentieth century, the family system was conceptualized as a whole, a totality different from the sum of the parts but yet with interrelated parts. The family unit was discussed as having a group psyche with certain identifiable types of interaction patterns. Scapegoating, rule-making and other types of small group patterns were identified and discussed as occurring within families. The unitary conceptualization of the family system is exemplified by the work of Smoyak (1975). The assumption is made that the whole affects the parts and vice versa, and that a problem with a part is reflective of a problem within the whole. The insistence of family therapists that the entire family be seen at one time in therapy sessions is reflective of this unitary concept.

The degree to which this is adhered varies with the individual therapy theory. When family system theories are examined for this unitary conceptualization, the question also arises, is the approach really unitary or is it merely a sum of the parts? A unitary approach seeks to understand the system, not individuals per se.

The second feature common to family systems theory is the assumption that there is an optimal functional state. Jackson's (1957) early work indicated that mental illness may serve to maintain the family or the homeostasis. Homeostasis in this instance has a negative connotation, but whether used in a positive or negative sense, the term means that the family system maintains a balance or steady state in which one factor balances the other. In the negative sense the schizophrenia of a child may hold together a strife-torn marital union. Later theorists, especially those influenced by the crises perspective, indicated that family equilibrium is a state to be regained after a disequilibrium-producing event. In the balancing of forces implied by equilibrium, a steady state is positive and is indicative of the optimal condition of the family system. Equilibrium in this sense implies a balance of forces within the family, a balance of roles, for example, within the family so as to counteract an upset state. When a parent dies, the family is sent into disequilibrium, in the crisis view, due to the loss of a member who performed many vital roles. As the family redistributes role functions, perhaps by reaching out to a support system in the community, equilibrium again may be reached.

If homeostasis is used to connote sameness or calmness as an optimal family quality, then the question needs to be asked, what occurs so that growth is possible within individual members and family as a group? When an adolescent child begins the individuation or breaking away process, for example, most families experience an upset in sameness and calmness. Yet growth of individual family members, most would agree, is necessary and unavoidable. A theory that seeks an optimal state of calmness (stasis) may not account for growth needs.

The term equilibrium utilized as an optimal state may or may not account for growth needs. Equilibrium as a state of rest attained by a counterbalance of forces is very similar to the homeostatic concept just described and probably will not account for growth. But if equilibrium is utilized in the sense of synchrony, then the term may account for growth processes. Synchrony, from the word synchrone, means to be joined in the same period but so that changing phases are possible. In other words, family members may grow, change, and develop within the family system. For example, the person who used to prepare meals may no longer perform this function because of an individual need, but within the family system, food may be available and prepared in some other manner. Thus, individual change (or growth) was possible and yet the family system remained intact.

Barnhill (1979), in a study of the optimal family system states discussed by most of the major family therapy theorists, presents eight dimensions of family health. These states are: individuation versus enmeshment; mutuality versus isolation; flexibility versus rigidity; stability versus disorganization; clear versus distorted perception; clear versus distorted communication; role reciprocity versus role conflict; and clear versus breached generational boundaries. Although there is a loss of specificity, these categories may be summarized to mean that the healthy family system is one which allows the full development of all members and yet remains a functional whole. In this idealized family, communication is clear (synchronous), generational boundaries are not breached because this would adversely affect individuation. The terms homeostasis and equilibrium if used to mean only a balance would not account for growth states. For example, enmeshment is a homeostatic state, whereas, individuation might cause upheaval and reformulation into a new form of family system.

It is possible to extrapolate primarily an open or closed system perspective from the various family systems theories. One way to describe the difference between closed and open systems is to use the discussion of meta models developed by Hultsch and Plemons (1979). The importance of this discussion to family systems theory has been identified by Fawcett (1980). There are two basic models utilized to define human beings and their relationship to the world around them—the organismic and the mechanistic models. The mechanistic model proposes cause and effect relationships. The machine is considered to be basically at rest until acted upon by some outside force. There is some time lag sequence implied as one waits for one part of the machine to affect the next. In this sense the machine is separate from the environmental field and additive in that the machine is the sum of the parts. The parts are very important in this model, for one part causes the next to function. The parts do not grow and change; patterns are repetitive. Machines (closed systems) do not take in extra stimuli, and unless the proper sequence of order is utilized to activate the machine, the machine will not function. For each machine action, there is a resultant reaction. For machines, processes are reversible, i.e., the whole procedure may be stopped and repeated in precisely the same manner and with little change in the machine. Machines in general do not regenerate, they wear down, wear out, and cease to function. Primarily linear in concept, machines close down, become entropic.

The organismic model according to Hultsch and Plemans is designed after a living organism and emphasizes wholeness; the parts are thus less important. Qualitative changes are possible within the organismic model (Hultsch and Plemons 1979, p. 5). Classical cause and effect relationships do not exist in the organismic model for with any given set of stimuli, the organism may act or not act in any given way. Living processes are not reversible in the sense that an organism progresses through time and space and is always growing older. The organismic model does not assume an at-rest state, rather this model assumes simultaneous activity, change, and growth (Hultsch and Plemons 1979). These theorists may be interpreted as positing that open systems are not repetitive and continuously patterned in the same way, that courses of action change. In systems terminology, living organisms display negentropy and equifinality. Each of the therapy theories chosen for discussion will be discussed in terms of unitary approach and conceptualization, assumption of optimal state, and a closed/open system perspective. These theories are then analyzed for reformulation utilizing specific nursing models.

SPECIFIC THERAPY APPROACHES
OF HALEY, MINUCHIN,
AND FRAMO   Haley, Minuchin, and Framo were chosen for this discussion because these theorists represent three distinct approaches to family therapy (Jones 1980). Haley, in his book *Problem Solving Therapy* (1978), states the basic concepts and propositions of his approach as it has evolved over time. It is important to note that, because Haley has written much and because his theoretical statements have changed over time, one of his latest theoretical works is used in this discussion. The approach of Haley in this work is unitary, not additive, for "to begin therapy by interviewing one person is to begin with a handicap" (Haley 1978, p. 10). Not only does Haley propose approaching the family as a unit, he emphasizes the need for discovering the social situation which makes the problem possible.

Some of the concepts of Haley are: the therapist, the field, family unit, family problem, directives, practice behavior, communication sequences, and communication hierarchy. Included as propositions are: the therapist becomes part of the field, or important to the family and influential in the situation before change can occur; therapy situations that are defined in terms of specific presenting problems are more amenable to change; it is the social situation, which displays a certain pattern and sequence, that makes the problem possible; assigned tasks solidify the gains of therapy as well as better illuminate the problem; change in communication sequences repatterns the behavior; and finally, secret coalitions across lines of authority produce confusion within the family system. Thus Haley is primarily concerned with the family as a unit and the interaction patterns which produce problems within the unit. The environment external to the family is considered important to the problem but not addressed at any length. An optimal family unit would be one in which there was a great diversity of response patterns, none of which deprived a member of his or her ability to grow and change (Haley 1978, p. 105).

Haley's approach indicates that he considers the family a living and somewhat open system that must accommodate growth needs. Although a few propositions, such as sequence of communication producing a problem situation, are cause/effect in nature, most propositions do not indicate classical cause/effect relationships. Haley states that in his approach the complexities of human life are simplified to reveal the structure, but that this is rather like describing a human being as a skeleton without flesh. Haley uses a few closed system terms such as control and resultant behavior. Haley's (1978) discussion of the drawback of family systems theories, i.e., steady state, equilibrium, not accounting for growth, is in essence a discussion of the drawbacks of a closed system model being applied to an open system, the family. The tasks or directives that Haley suggests are an effort to repattern the system. The tasks are expected to work directly and often call attention to an alternate pattern and at times emphasize a different aspect of the family system. The placing of emphasis on one aspect of the system in order to repattern may be understood as consistent with an open system approach. Thus, Haley's approach to the family indicates a sometimes open, sometimes closed system.

A hypothetical example of Haley's repatterning through the stages of therapy follows. This same example will be used throughout the chapter. The example is purposely made simplistic to emphasize differences in the approaches. It is important to note that any therapeutic approach would include much more than the simplistic steps identified in each example.

Although not specifically addressed here, the first session would have drawn out all family members as to their opinion of the problem. No interpretations would be made. A mother and father with a ten-year-old boy with cerebral palsy also have an eight-year-old boy who has developed night fears to such an extent he is afriad to fall asleep at night. The mother has been sleeping with this child to reassure him. The mother is intensely involved, however, with the care of the disabled child and the father works two jobs to raise more funds for the treatment of this child. Entering the family system through the parents, the therapist might approach disengagement of the mother from the over-involvement with the disabled child by assigning the father to assume the responsibility for reorganizing the care of the disabled child to include outside assistance. As the father has management skills, he might be directed to be the authority in an area in which he had been closed out. The therapist would be careful not to imply the mother has been incompetent, but rather acts in this manner to free her for other duties. The mother who has spent little time with the eight-year-old might be assigned to take this child out on several nights now that she is relieved of care, and spend the time talking with, enjoying, and getting to know the eight-year-old with enjoyable activities. The mother might also be directed to stop sleeping with this child and to have the father handle any problems or questions that arise in this matter. All of this initial process would be designed to involve the peripheral person, the father, in order to repattern the over-involvement of mother with the disabled child. Also, by entering the family system via parental concerns for the children, the therapist becomes central to the parents and thus engages them more fully in the therapy. By assigning tasks also, the therapist becomes part of the field for the period of time between sessions.

In the next phase of therapy, the parents might be encouraged to engage in adult activities by arranging time away from the children. At this step Haley might expect some resistance. The assumption would be that somehow the over-involvement of both parents is a means of keeping the parents separate. Any resistance to change might be dealt with perhaps by getting at anger between the two adults by discussing disparities. Perhaps the troubled marital relationship is related to feelings of despair and/or guilt over the disabled child. The child's night fears are assumed to be somehow connected to both stress in the marriage and the evening's sequence of events when the mother stays with the disabled child. This sequence has the effect of eliminating both the husband and also the eight-year-old child from involvement with the mother. The night fears might be thought to serve as some means of uniting the parents in the fearful child's room. Haley uses the identification of the sequence of events surrounding the behavior to illuminate the social situation that surrounds the problem. Unless the problem behavior ceases, however, Haley believes the therapy to be a failure.

It is important to note several things about Haley's approach. The family is assessed as a unit, not as a sum of parts, and there is no attempt to assess the individual's physical, social, and psychic needs. This individual assessment approach would contribute to continuance of the problem from the stages of therapy point of view. The family is approached as a dynamic unit, capable of change. An indirect manipulation via "directives" might be expected to result in a cause/effect result unless the therapist understands that several outcomes are possible from any directive. It is assumed in Haley's approach that optimal family functioning, i.e., more diverse patterns, would result from blocking the cross-generational coalitions. The intense involvement with the child on the part of the mother would be replaced with a joint new parental approach. The change and diversity that are sought eschew an equilibrium approach on the part of Haley.

Minuchin's approach in *Families and Family Therapy* (1974) indicates more of an open systems approach. Some of Minuchin's concepts are: family system, family structure, therapeutic system, and subsystems, or hierarchical groups of family members. Some of the propositions of Minuchin are: the individual is influenced by and influences constantly recurring sequences of interaction; an individual is reflective of the family system of which he is a part; stress in one part of the system affects other parts of the system; and changes in family structure contribute to changes in behavior of individuals within a given system.

Minuchin is primarily concerned with the family as a unit, not as a sum of individuals. Minuchin focuses more fully upon the contextual patterns operating within the unit. The optimal family functioning that Minuchin seeks to facilitate is flexible adaptation and the ability to restructure over time according to the demands of each new situation, keeping subsystem boundaries clear. This open system allows the members to grow and develop as needed. As with Haley, the emphasis is on present-day processes, not influences of the past. Although specificity is lost in a summary, the optimal family state for Minuchin is one which stresses flexibility, clear system boundaries, and growth needs of all members. Minuchin's model indicates an emphasis upon an open growing family system. Use of such phrases as "the therapist contributes to change" rather than "the therapist directs," indicates little cause/effect orientation. Although the assumption is made that changing the context will change the individual behavior, this change usually is not implied to be the one-to-one relationship of a closed system. Minuchin does state that when deviation goes beyond the systems tolerance, mechanisms are used by the family to re-establish equilibrium (Minuchin 1974, p. 52). His position is that the family must learn to adapt to change. Use of the term adaptation is not in the sense of an outside force acting upon the family, but rather a mutual change. A steady state or equilibrium is definitely not the goal, rather it is an evolving system with clear intra-system relationships that values the worth of the individual subsystems. The environment external to the family is not discussed in detail.

In the hypothetical situation that is simplified to emphasize differences, a Minuchin therapist would first attempt to join the family system for the purpose of engagement. By joining the system, the therapist experiences the context of the system and develops a "working diagnosis" (Minuchin 1974, p. 129). The therapist might join the system, through giving support, while the family discusses the problem. There is no attempt on the part of the therapist to assess individual physical, social, and psychic needs and no interpretations are made. The therapist tracks or asks clarifying questions about, for example, the sleeping arrangements and boundaries this family displays. The therapist might explore the parental systems functioning and the functioning of the sibling subsystem. During a first session the therapist evolves a "working diagnosis" similar to this: A non-functioning sibling subsystem is having difficulty operating effectively, and this is related to practically non-existent boundaries between the parental system and the child subsystem. The parental system is having difficulty functioning with several cross boundary problems.

The therapist in the initial session directs the participants to discuss the situation with each other; the children also are encouraged to discuss the issue that brought in the family. The therapist might thus illuminate the idiosyncratic system as well as recreate communication channels. Space might be changed and boundaries identified by sitting the children together. The children, with the help of the therapist, might agree to share a room at night. This arrangement would recognize that the youngest child is able to call for help if needed for the older child, and that the older child is thus able to assist with family functioning by serving as a companion to the younger child. The therapist thus might join the weak sibling subsystem supporting the boundaries. The therapist might also escalate stress by blocking the mother from verbally controlling the therapy session and also by emphasizing differences of opinion between the parents and children. Homework is sometimes assigned to be carried out, e.g., the parents might be asked to allow the children to handle the identified problem. This approach is to strengthen the sibling subsystem before working with the troubled parental system. Gradually, the therapist could move to a new area, e.g., the parents' troubled marital union.

Although the system is in a sense manipulated, Minuchin points out that any task given may elicit any number of responses. The responses, however, tend to expand the family's repertoire and hence tend to be change enhancing. Although identification of boundaries seems inflexible in a change model, Minuchin perceives boundaries as harmonious with functioning systems.

Framo's approach in *Rationale and Techniques of Intensive Family Therapy* (1965) also demonstrates a unitary approach to the family system. However, terms indicative more of a closed system perspective seem clearer. Some of Framo's concepts are: family system, past unresolved problems, family rules, resistance, and transference. Some derived propositions of Framo are: the therapist must stop old patterns before change can occur; rules hold the family in a repetitious cycle; past unresolved problems tend to be acted out in the present family; the attachment of past feelings to present family members tends to hold the family in a repetitive cycle; and accumulated experiences with present family members and the mutual accommodations made to these experiences tend to account for present behaviors.

Framo is primarily concerned with the family as an operating system or unit. The focus is on the psychodynamics and resultant behavior. The goal of therapy or the optimal system state is a clear perception by members of one another, as free as possible from past influences and misperceptions. The emphasis is more upon the past affecting the present. Framo's approach is primarily a closed system perspective for the family therapy addresses past problems. It can be interpreted that the family will remain enmeshed unless acted upon by some outside force. Since the family rules hold the family in a state of equilibrium, the goal of therapy is to establish a new equilibrium based upon accurate perceptions of the here and now. The environment external to the family is not addressed to any great extent.

In the hypothetical situation, a Framo approach would take place over time. The family would need to agree to work over time with the therapist. The family also must be willing to bring into the therapy sessions any extended family members identified as essential to the primary family unit (Framo 1965, p. 147). Several evaluation sessions are held to determine underlying situations. The initial presented problem is rarely thought to be indicative of the underlying situation. The family is asked to identify the changes they would like to occur. In the simplified example, family members, including the child with cerebral palsy, would be asked to discuss their version of the problem and this would assist with identifying transactional patterns. The parents would be encouraged to discuss their feelings regarding their families of origin, as well as events in their early and present marriage. The therapist thus works to clarify feelings regarding the past, thereby assisting the parents to gain some insight. The therapist might confront the mother with her absenting behavior in terms of the marital relationship and make some interpretation in this regard. Perhaps anger is related to some past event or perhaps some anger at their families of origin.

The therapist at the end of several evaluation sessions develops his or her diagnosis: there are coalition patterns, e.g., between the mother and the disabled child; there are family myths, e.g., that the relationship problems occur because of the disabled child; and that the fearful child's acting out is somehow related to holding the family together. During the middle phase of therapy, the therapist would most likely focus on working through feelings and working out new relationship patterns. The therapist would be careful not to perpetuate the family system status quo. According to Framo, resistance to change is expected and must be identified and challenged. In the final or termination phase of therapy, the attempt is to solidify gains. In the optimal case, the parents would be better able to discuss feelings openly and decrease the overinvolvement with the children. The children are thus free to pursue their own interests. Resistance to termination might be encountered, e.g., the "well" sibling (the disabled child) and later the index child (the fearful child) might act out their separation and dissolution fears. Termination issues are handled directly and the family should be freer to relate on the basis of present reality to one another.

The family system in this view is seen as repetitive, and entropic in its initial state. Changing the family by breaking the old rules or equilibrium and establishing a new relational system is the goal. The internal environment of the family is of prime importance and the family is approached without much utilization of the external environment. Physic processes are important and related to the system problems.

CORRELATES OF PERSON, HEALTH, ENVIRONMENT, AND NURSING WITHIN THE
THERAPY MODELS AND THE NURSING MODELS   In Haley's model, the person is seen as part of the total family system, a subsystem, as it were, whose behavior is understandable in terms of the whole family system. Health in Haley's schema is the ability to change, grow, and develop a repertoire of diverse ways of handling life situations (1978, p. 105). The environment external to the family is not addressed although Haley identifies that external events should be considered. The therapist (or nurse) in Haley's model is a participant in the system but is also a director, in control of the therapy.

In Minuchin's model the person is understood in terms of the total family system. Behavior, although not totally predictable, is understandable primarily in terms of family system functioning. Extrapolated, health is the ability to grow, change, develop, and function as a member of the family system. The environment external to the family affects the family, such as economic depression. The nature of the relationship to environment is not, however, addressed at any length. The nurse (or therapist) in Minuchin's model would be much less the director, but more of a facilitator of repatterning within the context of the system.

In Framo's model, the person is more influenced by past situations that affect the present family system. Health is interpreted as the freedom from past experience so as to live more fully in the present with clearer perceptions. Environment external to the primary and extended family is not generally considered. In all of the above family therapy theories, person, health, and environment are viewed in light of psychosocial considerations. Physical or biological considerations are not usually addressed.

The therapist-nurse in Haley's model would be more of an active director who assigns tasks. At times, to influence change in the family system, paradoxical injunctions might be given. The therapist-nurse in Minuchin's model is also an active participant within the system. Not in control but rather participating and influencing, the therapist joins this system and might attempt to escalate stress in the system so as to facilitate change. A therapist-nurse in Framo's model is more of an evaluator, analyzer, and a reflector. The therapist-nurse might at various times clarify, confront, and support as new patterns are worked out.

In Rogers' (1980) conceptual model, the study of the environmental field is considered integral with the study of person (man in her terminology). In contrast, all three family therapists discuss that the individual can only be understood in his or her context—the family system. Man according to Rogers is conceived of as a four-dimensional energy field embedded in a four-dimensional environmental field. Rogers conceives of man as an indivisible unit—by studying only an individual's biology, for example, one cannot know the whole person. Man as a four-dimensional energy field manifests openness, or negentropy and pattern and organization. The environment is also a four-dimensional negentropic energy field characterized by pattern and organization; environment encompasses all that is outside the human field (Rogers 1980, p. 332). Thus it seems that Rogers would consider the family, although not specifically addressed, a negentropic energy field embedded in the larger environmental field. Nursing as a verb is seen as working with the energy field, not for or on the client (Falco and Lobo 1980, p. 173). The nurse is part of the co-extensive energy field, not separate. Health, although not addressed specifically, may be extrapolated as symphonic interactions between persons and their environment, a coherence and integrity of the human field (Falco and Lobo

1980). Rogers' conceptual model requires consideration of development, or unidirectional change in her words. That is, since each person is progressing (or developing) in one direction only, this progression must be accounted for in the interaction pattern of the energy field.

Roy's conceptual framework views person as a biophychosocial being (Roy 1980). Roy states persons are also related to others in the group (Roy 1980, p. 3). The person as a whole should be viewed therefore from biologic/psychologic and social science perspectives. It is unclear if the biopsychosocial parts are assessed separately and from this, knowledge is applied to the adaptive modes, or if the sum of the parts can never equal the whole. It seems that environment is all that is external to the person. Health is considered an inevitable dimension of life and extrapolated health is optimal adaptation or high level wellness on the health-illness continuum (Roy 1976). The goal is to maintain the integrity of the whole. Roy discusses developmental processes, developmental stages, and crises. The nurse as a person external to the client evaluates and determines whether the individual is experiencing an adaptation problem or is in need of additional assistance. The nurse might then assist the family to adapt more fully or to change the nature of the focal stimulus so that it falls within the adaptive range. The person, although in constant interaction with his environment, seems to be the prime focus; family is not addressed in great length.

Orem's model views person (man in her terminology) as a psychophysiologic organism with rational powers (Calley, et al. 1980, p. 303). Nursing gives direct assistance to those unable to meet their own self-care needs. Health is a state of wholeness or integrity of the individual human being, his parts, and his modes of functioning (Orem 1980, Foster and Janssens 1980). Orem states that man's functioning is linked to his environment (Orem 1971). It would seem that environment is all that is external to the person. Orem, in an interesting discussion of the way family is to be approached, suggests that within the concept of wholeness, families are important. However, the parts (individual members) have existence and operations apart from the whole and, it would seem, must be assessed separately. Orem suggests that the nursing of families requires a special knowledge base different from, yet complementary to, that of individuals alone. It would seem that congruence between Orem's model and a family systems theory might be approached from her nursing systems perspective. That is, nursing systems are formed when nurses use their abilities to provide for groups by performing systems of action.

Congruence and Reformulation Issues
It is important that nursing as a discipline reformulate, according to its purposes and needs, the theories derived from other fields

(Fawcett 1978, Kaplan 1963). The issue is that a discipline changes, adapts, and reformulates for its purposes, extant concepts, and groups of concepts. In this section the nursing models are utilized to reformulate selected aspects of the above family system theories. The family systems theory of Haley is compared to Orem's model and needed reformulations are addressed. Both Haley and Orem are considered to utilize both mechanistic and organismic concepts. The assumption is made in terms of both theorists of sometimes open, sometimes closed systems. Orem identifies that an important first step in nursing care is the diagnosis or identification of the problem. This is quite similar to Haley's insistence upon definition of the family problem in terms of a specific behavior. Orem's way of arriving at the problem statement is to assess: (1) what is the self-care demand (what is the problem); (2) does the patient have a deficit for engaging in self-care (what are the abilities of family members to handle the problem); (3) what is the reason for the problem's existence (what is the relationship of subsystems, the hierarchical sequence that makes the problem possible); (4) should the patient be helped to refrain from self-care (is the family system capable of participating in the therapy, or must the nurse therapist temporarily direct and control); and (5) what is the patient's potential for engaging in self-care (what is the optimal functioning that can be expected of this family system in relation to the problem) (Orem 1980, p. 203).

The most evident areas of congruence between Haley and Orem deal with the therapist (nurse) as the director of therapy. Orem states that step one in the nursing process is determining why the patient is under care (see above diagnostic steps). Step two is to design a system of nursing that will contribute to the goals. If the goal is to change a problematic family behavior, the nurse identifies changes that are needed in roles and resources, for example, and identifies the approach so that the changes might be most effective. This is similar to Haley's concept of giving specific directives to the family that involve details in terms of time and specific frequencies. Whereas Orem seems to indicate that the nurse is separate during assessment, this could be interpreted as using much the same approach as Haley, i.e., the care giver experiences the context and then, as it were, steps back and directs. In the final step of the nursing process, the caregiver, according to Orem, compensates for self-care deficits, overcomes self-care limitations, and fosters and protects self-care abilities and limitations. This might be interpreted as an area of difference between Haley and Orem. In this last step Orem could be interpreted to indicate that environmental resources might be utilized to overcome any inherent deficits. Haley does not deal with the environment to any great extent.

In the hypothetical situation presented, these differences between Haley and Orem are apparent. That is, a community agency, such as

Crippled Children's Commission, might be employed to take over some of the financial burden felt by the father. Self-care limitations might be overcome by utilizing some ongoing community resource such as homemaking service to free the mother from some of her duties. The father and mother thus would be freer to function as marriage partners. In the areas of fostering and protecting development, an Orem therapist would recognize that the fearful child's development might be limited or thwarted in terms of allowing him to learn to care for himself by the overprotection of his mother. The Orem therapist might identify the disabled child as a self-care resource within the family and thus suggest, after discussions, that both children sleep in the same room, thus assisting one another. In terms of fostering self-care and protecting the self-care abilities, it seems that an Orem therapist would not insist on termination within a specified number of sessions as Haley does. Recognizing that the newly established family self-care system needs support, some sort of continuing assistance would be offered for continuity of care.

Two other points of disparity between Orem and Haley are that Orem indicates that family collaboration and physical needs should be considered. Orem states that the family's interest or ability to collaborate in care must be assessed (Orem 1980, p. 204). In other words, an Orem therapist would consider reviewing the plan for therapy with the family, rather than using a non-informed manipulation approach. Orem states that meeting the immediate self-care need is a first step towards collaboration and/or participation in family self-care. Once the family is functioning so that a state of wellness of the family system is near, then collaboration and participation in self-care would definitely be addressed. It thus might be reviewed with the family that the child's fears were related to the family's pattern of coping, that the closeness of the mother with the children, although designed to help them, was not allowing for the growth and assumption of responsibility of which the children were capable. It would also be reviewed with the parents that friction between them is always felt in the system and that direct discussion of differences between the parents is necessary. An Orem therapist might temporarily give directives and control, but at some later point the family would be enlisted as collaborators.

In terms of the physical needs, Orem sees man as a psychophysiologic organism, as a biologic organism in an environment with physical and biologic components (Calley et al. 1980). As such, an Orem therapist would recognize that physiologic responses, such as gastrointestinal problems of the fearful child, have a psychological aspect. Therefore, the therapist would consider these GI problems as secondary to the family system problem. The nurse therapist, however, would assess the physical state of all the members, realizing that just as the mind may affect the body, the opposite is also true.

The family systems theory of Framo (1965) is compared to Roy's (1976) model and reformulations are addressed. Both Roy and Framo utilize more mechanistic than organismic concepts. Assumptions appear to be made that the family is sometimes a closed and sometimes an open system. Although Roy does not discuss the family as a system to any great extent, her consideration of the whole person with his or her total environment, as well as insistence upon considering the developmental state of the person, leads one to conclude that, within her model, the family system should be considered.

Galbreath (1980 p. 206) discusses Roy's model and the family system. She refers to Boszormenyi-Nagy, an associate of Framo. The reference is to the way in which an enmeshed (or closed) family system, keeps a child from individuation. The parent adapts to a focal stimulus, a need for companionship, by disallowing the child to separate. This is considered a case of maladaptation in terms of the system because the child's developmental needs are stifled and hence his or her integrity is threatened. A central concept in Roy's model (1976, p. 3), adaptation, is discussed as being carried out in the physiological, self concept, role function, and interdependence modes. Adaptation is thought to occur within an acceptable range; a response outside of this range is considered maladaptive.

If one considered the family system to incorporate the above modes, the concept of adaptation as utilized by Roy might be applied quite readily. For example, family systems have physiologic needs such as food, clothing, and shelter. As part of this need, it is necessary that the family provide adequate amounts and types of these supplies. An overcrowded family, for example, might lead to problems in one of the adaptation modes. Family systems have self-concept needs, both of the family subsystems, or individuals, and the family as a whole. An inadequate self-concept on the part of the parent might lead the parent to adapt by utilizing his or her children, over whom he or she has more control, as life companions. A deficit in the parent's self-concept would be hypothesized in terms that the parent views himself or herself as inadequate in terms of relating to adults. This child companionship thus would eliminate the need to seek other adult companions who might find the adult wanting. This turning inward would lead to an enmeshed or closed down family. Such families are described by both Framo (1965) and Boszormenyi-Nagy (1965).

Role function needs and interdependence needs might be seen as leading to maladaption within the hypothetical family system. Every family has a number of roles that must be fulfilled such as child caregiver, fund raiser, companion, etc. When these roles are not fulfilled, role conflict occurs and maladaptation may result, i.e., the integrity of the system is threatened. In the hypothetical situation, the role of care-giver to the disabled child was superceding all other roles. The roles such as mother of the fearful child, marital partner, and adult were not being handled and interdependence maladaption existed in the sense that the children were not allowed to separate from the parents.

Intervention in Roy's model is the key to nursing activity; the nurse changes the perceived parental inadequacy by manipulating the environment by increasing, decreasing, removing, or altering stimuli (Galbreath 1980). The person is seen basically in an "at rest" state, and the nurse is seen as the operator, altering the input stimuli. These relationships suggest a mechanistic view.

In Framo's approach to the hypothetical family, the parents may be seen as living out past problems in terms of the present family. In other words, there are definite problems with self-concept. By manipulating the environment, the stimuli is altered; that is, by allowing the parents to ventilate, and work through their past feelings in the present therapy sessions, the self-concept changes and the perceptions are brought into normal range. These relationships also suggest a closed system conceptualization.

A Roy approach to the family system would include assessment of the various adaptive modes. A deficit would be found in the role function, self-concept, and interdependence modes. It is doubtful that the intervention would include only a catharsis. A nurse therapist approaching the family from the Roy model likely would utilize the environment. The parents would be separated from the children. The space in the home probably would also be assessed in terms of the children's sleeping arrangements and be changed to facilitate the care. Because of Roy's emphasis upon developmental stages, the children and parents would be encouraged to individuate with support and find companions in their own age group. Other developmental tasks would be assessed and addressed.

Because of Roy's emphasis on physiologic adaptation, the physiologic needs of the members would be addressed. Roy's approach to the family system would therefore be more comprehensive with more attention to other environmental factors than that of Framo. In the interventions identified by Roy (1980), there is emphasis on teaching and educating the patient; most likely the family would be taught what were the bases of their problem. Roy suggests with dysfunctional interdependence modes that cognitive and affective structuring may be changed through insight therapy (1976, p. 392). Insight therapy is of course related to Framo's approach. Outlets for the parents would be identified to decrease temporary spillover of tension onto the children.

The manipulation of the environment is encouraged to provide for independence as congruent as possible with developmental level.

Because of similarities, the structural family theory of Minuchin is compared with Rogers' conceptual framework. Both are considered primarily open systems approaches. Reformulations are addressed and the reformulated model is used to analyze the hypothetical situation. The areas of similarity between Minuchin and Rogers have to do with Minuchin's field approach. Energy fields extend to infinity (Rogers 1980) and in Minuchin's model, the contextual field of the family, as well as the extended field, is the unit of analysis. Rogers is interpreted to extend this to mean that the family may be conceived of as an energy field. The family field is considered in Minuchin's structural theory to be greater and different from the sum of the parts or the individuals. Otherwise, Minuchin would assess the parts or individuals separately rather than in interaction; this is not the case. The approach to the whole rather than parts is an area of congruence with Rogers. In Rogers' conceptualization, energy fields are always open. Minuchin's view that the family is a system that must change and grow according to internal and external forces would seem compatible with Rogers. Openness in Minuchin's terms is related to the constantly evolving patterns that are never entirely predictable.

Pattern and organization identify energy fields (Rogers 1980); patterns and organization also are continuously changing. In part, Minuchin's position that the family system must account for changing requirements is a recognition of this continuous change. As children grow, the family system is repatterned. Adults in Minuchin's view also grow and change and these simultaneous events account for the dynamic nature of the family system. Just as the family system continuously grows, changes, and repatterns, Minuchin indicates and Rogers stresses that so also does the environment. The environment is, in Rogers' conceptual model, an energy field, a system that grows, changes, evolves, and repatterns. The fluctuations in weather patterns are examples of this change as well as fluctuating patterns manifested in the development of towns and cities. Rogers' concepts seem compatible with Minuchin for he specifically addresses the repatterning of the economic system—economic depression—as one pattern that affects the family. The point made by Rogers is that she considers the effect of the environmental field upon the family to be, not one of cause and effect, but rather one of mutual interaction. This position would seem fairly compatible with Minuchin. The therapist in influencing the family system never directly controls the situation. Rogers' principle of helicy postulates that change is continual, innovative, probabilistic, and characterized by increasing diversity (Rogers 1970, 1980). Minuchin's approach can be interpreted as identifying the need to handle change although this is less true than with Rogers. When Minuchin states one "works with" the system, this might be interpreted to mean that change is innovative and probabilistic rather than cause and effect. In other words, although all adolescents come to individuation, the general pattern is there, no two adolescents separate from the family in quite the same way. The situation probably has certain features, the fearful parent, the rejecting adolescent—but none of this is certain.

Rogers further postulates that the human and environmental fields are characterized by resonancy. That is, wave patterns manifest change from longer waves, lower frequency to higher frequency shorter waves. One might postulate that each family member manifests different field patterns and that the entire family thus manifests some diverse yet unified pattern. The environmental field also manifests a diverse yet whole pattern. Perhaps Minuchin's approach to synchronous subsystem boundaries is an attempt to effect a synchrony between and among the various system patterns. But just as there is no cause/effect in Rogers' approach, Minuchin's approach can be interpreted to indicate the therapist attempts repatterning, not that repatterning is caused to happen. Minuchin emphasizes that only by working with the family system will individual patterns change.

Minuchin's concept of working within the context of the family can be interpreted in a Rogerian sense, i.e., that the total field context or family system is an influential force in terms of the individual field. With both Rogers and Minuchin, the whole is most important and approaches are nonadditive, change models.

Rogers' third principle is complementarity or that interaction between human and environmental fields is continuous, simultaneous, and mutual. A corollary of the principle is that there is no separation between man and environment. Minuchin's concept of boundaries seems incongruent with both resonancy and complementarity. That is, if fields extend to infinity and are in mutual simultaneous interaction, then there are no boundaries. Rogers does state, however, that use of the term boundaries is acceptable to aid perception. The human ability to perceive fields is very limited and what seems to be a boundary may in essence be a different field pattern. What Minuchin refers to as marking boundaries may be effecting a decrease in the invasive repatterning of one field by another.

Other terms of Minuchin, such as adaptation, stress, and equilibrium, also need to be changed or deleted in light of Rogers' model. If adaptation means the process of accommodating to some outside force from a state of rest, then this concept would be incongruent with Rogers' position. Minuchin, however, states that by facilitating the use of alternative modes, the therapist makes use of the family matrix (field) in the process of healing (facilitating synchrony). This interpretation would be acceptable in Rogers' terms. However, Minuchin goes on to say that the family structure must be able to adapt. As previously discussed, this implies a closed system perspective and needs to be changed. The continued existence of the family as a system depends on a sufficient range of patterns, availability of alternative patterns, and flexibility to mobilize as necessary. This is an area of congruence for both theorists. Minuchin's approach could be reformulated to mean that, in a particular family system, the greater the range of complex patterns available for the subsystem, the more likely the total field is to exhibit synchrony.

Rogers' definition of health, as extrapolated from Newman (1979), is symphonic interaction between persons and their environment, a coherence. An invasive field that, in effect, attempts to repattern another according to its own needs, is not a coherent force within the family unit. Thus cross-generational coalitions inhibit the development and change of the less developed unit. Perhaps the more established field of the adult is one of more intensity, and if a coalition develops, the newer evolving field may not develop its own pattern. Minuchin's extrapolated definition of health is flexible adaptation and the ability to restructure over time according to the demands of each new situation. Flexible adaptation might be reformulated to non-invasive synchrony between field forces within the family system.

In the hypothetical situation, a reformulated structural approach might be relabeled to indicate less of a mechanistic nature. In the reformulated theory, the nurse using Rogers' model might approach the hypothetical situation differently. Because in the example the family unit is composed of several members, the nurse would seek to identify the points of disharmony within the field. The fearful child is symptomatic of family disharmony. The nurse, as part of the environmental field, seeks to promote synchromy and development of emergent field patterns by influencing the family field towards a more synchronous patterning. Recognizing the dysynchrony related to invasive closeness of one field (the mother) with another field (that of the child with cerebral palsy), the nurse seeks to influence the repatterning of this relationship. The fears of the other child are considered to be a manifestation of a field which is in distress. Part of the disharmony of the family field is related to the absence of the father, or at least disparity of approach between the mother and the father. The nurse, in assessing the situation, might attempt to experience the family system or field using all of her senses and skills.

Any attempt at repatterning would be developed with the family and addressed as attempts at reformulating or trying out a new pattern. Although the Rogers' approach might parallel Minuchin's in the hypothetical situation in many ways, the differences would revolve around working with the family, not manipulating, not by identifying boundaries, but by identifying the different growth patterns and needs. Placing the children in the same bedroom is an example of an attempt to synchronize fields of similar frequency.

The physical needs of the family members are considered as manifestations of the total field. Consequently these are addressed if disharmony is evident. But, rather than addressed as a separate entity, the needs are looked upon as manifestations of the whole. The child with cerebral palsy may be quite healthy and display little physical disharmony, whereas the fearful child may display some type of physical disharmony, such as dietary and gastrointestinal problems. Thus, parts of individual subsystems may be addressed but always considered in terms of the whole. In a particulate approach, gastrointestinal problems of the fearful child would be treated alone, and probably with little success as separate from the total family field.

RESEARCH AND PRACTICE
ISSUES   Although all three reformulated models are quite different, there are common elements. These commonalities have to do with approaching assessment from a holistic stance. That is, the psychic state of health of a family or individual is not the total focus in the reformulated nursing approach, whereas many of the family therapy theories utilize a psychic assessment approach only. The nursing therapies focus more broadly; a recognition is made that, for example, a mother with severe iron deficiency anemia may very well handle her fatigue by interacting with a parental child. A second area of commonality is that the nursing therapy approaches deal with family/individual participation. Most of the nursing models eschew a silent manipulation as the nurse assesses and treats; all the models suggest an openness with clients. That is, the silent, never revealed manipulation of the system is not the approach indicated by the nursing models. Roy, for example, states that environmental manipulation must be approached, and attempts to solidify gains through teaching and other explanatory attempts. The family or client is seen as active, more as a partner in therapy rather than in the passive sick role posture. Even Minuchin, who is relatively open with families, does not share with them what he believes to be the underlying situation. Finally, the nursing therapies, when compared to some other therapy theories, seem an optimistic approach. The family is not seen as totally foretold by past family systems, living out past echoes as it were. The family is conceived of as primarily healthy or tending toward health and capable of learning, growing, and changing as completely as needed. The nursing approach

therefore includes discussing with the family the patterns that are seen as dysfunctional, and working with the family utilizing strengths to change these patterns and interrelationships. Because the deep-seated, intractable, and pathology-laden interpretations of the family dysfunction are not made, the traditional loathing to share the diagnosis of the underlying problems with the family is less.

The research and practice issues in a sense revolve around the reformulations. Not many of the therapy theories have been systematically explored in terms of outcomes (Wells et al. 1978). Rather than address outcome evaluation, which all therapy theories need to do, some of the research issues that revolve around the reformulated nursing therapy approaches will be addressed. With the Rogers approach, there are several basic and applied questions:

Is family dysfunction an invasiveness of one field force with another?

If family health is synchrony, how is repatterning best accomplished?

Is there a family energy field that may be considered in relation to other energy fields?

There are many more research issues that may be readily identified.

In a reformulation with Orem's model, some research issues might be:

What is the nature of a total family assessment that also includes individual data?

How does one maintain a family perspective using individual assessment data?

How does one assess a family self-care deficit?

What is the nature of family self-care agency, etc.?

Orem discusses that the nursing of groups requires a specialized knowledge base. The nature of the knowledge base most complimentary with an Orem approach should be explored.

In a reformulation with Roy's model, there are several research issues that might be addressed:

Do the adaptation modes transfer readily to the family system?

Is family health an additive concept comprised of individual assessments?

Does one assess family adaptation modes and then only intervene in the stimuli?

The practice issues flow from the theoretical reformulations.

The effect of educating the family to the underlying problem also needs to be assessed. The traditional individual psychoanalytic approach held that teaching and education were of little value. The troubling situation had to be relived and experienced before insight and resolution could result. If a Roy approach incorporates both education and insight goals, then the relationship of education to insight needs to be addressed. The traditional view is that after insight, little education is needed. Another important issue in the Roy approach has to do with manipulation of the external environment, and whether this is effective when dealing with the family unit.

The above reformulated nursing therapy approaches are a first attempt to accomplish what Kaplan (1963) and Fawcett (1978) indicate lies before us. That is, rather than borrowing in total extant family theories, nursing must reformulate to its own purposes. Some might question the effect of nurse therapists practicing from a variety of approaches, but, after all this is currently the case, for nurses are practicing using a multiplicity of unchanged theories.

References

Ackerman N: Prejudice and scapegoating in the family. *In* Zuk G, Boszormenyi-Nagy I (Eds.): Family Therapy and Disturbed Families, Palo Alto, Science & Behavior Books, 1967

Barnhill L: Healthy family systems. Fam Coordinator, (January), 94–100, 1979

Boszormenyi-Nagy I: A theory of relationships: experience and transaction. *In* Boszormenyi-Nagy I, Framo J (Eds.): Intensive Family Therapy: Theoretical and Practical Aspects, New York, Harper & Row, 1965

Broderick C: Beyond the five conceptual frameworks: a decade of development in family theory. J Marriage and the Family, 33:139–159, 1971

Calley J, Dirksen M, Engalla M, Hennrich M: The Orem self-care nursing model. *In* Riehl J, Roy C: Conceptual Models for Nursing Practice (2nd Ed.), New York, Appleton-Century-Crofts, 1980

Donaldson S, Crowley D: The discipline of nursing. Nurs Outlook, 26:113–120, 1978

Falco S, Lobo M: Martha E. Rogers. In the Nursing Theories Conference Group. Nursing Theories: The Base for Professional Nursing Practice. Englewood Cliffs, Prentice-Hall, 1980

Fawcett J: The "what" of theory development. *In* Theory Development: What, Why, How? New York, National League for Nursing, 1978

Fawcett J: Address to a nursing doctoral seminar on family health, May 14, 1980. Jacqueline Fawcett, PhD, RN, is an Associate Professor, School of Nursing, University of Pennsylvania

Foster P, Janssens N: Dorothy E. Orem. In the Nursing Theories Conference Group. Nursing Theories: The Base for Professional Nursing Practice. Englewood Cliffs, Prentice-Hall, 1980

Framo J: Rationale and techniques of intensive family therapy. *In* Boszormenyi-Nagy I, Framo J (Eds.): Intensive Family Therapy: Theoretical & Practical Aspects, New York. Harper & Row, 1965

Galbreath J: Sister Callista Roy. In the Nursing Theories Conference Group. Nursing Theories: The Base for Professional Nursing Practice, Englewood Cliffs, Prentice-Hall, 1980

Haley J: The family of the schizophrenic: a model system. J Nervous and Mental Disorders, 129:357–374, 1959

Haley J: Problem Solving Therapy, San Francisco, Jossey Bass, 1978

Hill R: Families Under Stress. New York, Harper & Row 1949

Hill R: Modern systems theory and the family: a confrontation. *In* Sussman M: Sourcebook in Marriage and the Family, Boston, Houghton-Mifflin Company, 1974

Hill R, Hansen D: The identification of conceptual frameworks utilized in family study. Marriage and Family Living, 22:299–301, 1960

Hill R, Katz A, Simpson R: An inventory of research in marriage and family behavior: a statement of objectives and progress. Marriage & Family Living, 19:89–92, 1957

Hultsch D, Plemons J: Life events and life-span development. *In* Baltes P, Brim O (Eds.): Life Span Development and Behavior, Vol. 2, New York, Academic Press, 1979

Jackson D: The question of family homeostasis. Psychiatric Quarterly Supplement, 31:79–90, 1957

Jones S: Family Therapy: A Comparison of Approaches, Bowie, Maryland, Robert J. Brady Co., 1980

Kaplan A: The Conduct of Inquiry, New York, Harper & Row, 1963

Lindemann E: Symptomatology and management of acute grief. Am J Psych, 101:141–148, 1944

Minuchin S: Families and Family Therapy. Cambridge, Harvard University Press, 1974

Napier A, Whitaker C: The Family Crucible, New York, Harper & Row, 1978

Newman M: Theory Development in Nursing, Philadelphia, F. A. Davis, 1979

Nye F, Berardo F: Emerging Conceptual Frameworks in Family Analysis, New York, The Macmillan Company, 1966

Orem D: Nursing: Concepts of Practice (2nd ed.), New York, McGraw-Hill, 1980

Parad H, Caplan G: A framework for studying families in crises. Social Work, 5:3–15, 1960

Rogers M: An Introduction to the Theoretical Basis of Nursing, Philadelphia, F. A. Davis, 1970

Rogers M: Nursing: a science of unitary man. *In* Riehl J, Roy C (Eds.): Conceptual Models for Nursing Practice, New York, Appleton-Century-Crofts, 1980

Roy C: The Roy adaptation model. *In* Riehl J, Roy C (Eds.): Conceptual Models for Nursing Practice, New York, Appleton-Century-Crofts, 1980

Smoyak S: Introducing families to family therapy. *In* Smoyak S (Ed.): The Psychiatric Nurse as a Family Therapist, New York, J. Wiley, 1975

Wells R, Dilkes T, Trivelli N: The results of family therapy: a critical review of the literature. Family Process, 7:189–207, 1972

Whall A: Congruence between family theory and nursing models. Adv Nurs Sci, 3:59–67, 1980

5 RHYTHM THEORY: RELATIONSHIP TO NURSING CONCEPTUAL MODELS

Judith A. Floyd

Within psychiatric mental health nursing, the importance of a theoretical basis for practice has been recognized for some time (Muller 1950, Peplau 1952). Psychiatric mental health nurses have continually explored the contributions of theories developed within other disciplines and found a number of theories useful in organizing empirical findings in the field of mental health. At the same time, psychiatric mental health nurses have noted that theories developed within other disciplines do not reflect the unique perspective of nursing. A number of authors have attempted to describe how the practice of psychiatric mental health nurses differs from the practice of other professionals in the mental health field (Fagin 1967, Lego 1973, Mellow 1968; Ujhely 1973). Each has attempted to adapt theories developed within the conceptual systems of other disciplines to his own conceptualization of nursing.

A logical way to continue the development of theory relevant to psychiatric mental health nursing practice is to reformulate existing theory within the major nursing conceptual models. One advantage of attempting reformulations within these well-known models is that such conceptual models have been subject to continual development through critique and debate. In addition, the utilization of familiar nursing conceptual models increases the potential for an interchange of ideas with nursing colleagues in other specialty areas of nursing.

At the present time, nursing's conceptual system has evolved to the point where there is general consensus regarding the central concepts basic to any conceptual model of nursing: person, environment, health, and nursing. Scholars of the major conceptual models of nursing have noted that each model addresses the nature of the person-environment interaction and the relationship of this interaction to health and illness (Fawcett 1980, Flaskerud and Holleran 1980, Whall 1980).

In the development of nursing models, the person is often described as a biopsychosocial being in order to capture the holistic nature of the person-environment interaction. It is not surprising, therefore, that attempts within nursing to reformulate theories have utilized theories developed primarily within the conceptual systems of biology, psychology, and sociology.

Within psychiatric mental health nursing, attempts to reformulate existing and developing theories have drawn primarily from psychological and sociological theories which directly illuminate the nature of mental health and illness. However, some attempts at reformulation have also drawn from the fields of biology, anthropology, and philosophy (Auger 1973, Leininger 1973, Osborne 1973, Paterson and Zderad 1976, Pothier 1978, Sayre 1978, Stephens 1976). As the understanding of the holistic nature of person-environment interaction develops, the reformulation of theory from a very broad range of disciplines will make a contribution to theory development in psychiatric mental health nursing.

This chapter focuses on the reformulation of rhythm theory, a major contribution from biology. The nursing conceptual models used for the reformulation are those proposed by Rogers (1970, 1980) and Newman (1979). A nursing conceptual model that is to be used as an organizing network for a reformulation of rhythm theory should be an open systems model. Continuous rhythmic activity in system variables is inconsistent with the laws of closed systems. Rhythmic activity would be excluded from human behavior if the laws of closed systems were strictly applied to human systems. However, being open systems, living organizations can occupy states considerably displaced from equilibrium. One of the prominent features of these states is the occurrence of rhythmic activity. Since Rogers' conceptual model emphasizes system openness and the rhythmic nature of person-environment interaction (Rogers 1970, 1980), her conceptual model is utilized. Newman's conceptual model of health (Newman 1979) is also utilized since it, too, is based on an open systems view of person-environment interaction.

THE RHYTHM PERSPECTIVE   Although "rhythm theory" was referred to in the introduction as an existing theory, there is to date no unified theory of rhythmic phenomena. There is, however, a rhythm perspective generated by the research and theory building efforts of scholars from many disciplines. The variety of rhythmic phenomena studied in humans includes very short rhythms such as brain waves or heart rhythms, as well as very long rhythms such as the life-span cycle. In between these two extremes are rhythms of varying length such as the daily rhythms of body temperature, urinary output, and sleep, the monthly menstrual cycle, and the childbearing year. A number of environmental rhythms have also been studied, most notably light and darkness, tidal movements, and changes.

A general vocabulary has evolved as rhythm researchers from

many disciplines have sought to communicate with one another. The basic terms defined here are extrapolated from the definitions developed by Aschoff (1965), Conroy and Mills (1970), and Sollberger (1965). An understanding of this terminology is basic to determining in what ways concepts and relationships from the rhythm framework may need to be reformulated to be consistent with Rogers and Newman's conceptual models.

The term *rhythm* is used to indicate the recurrence of similar processes at similar intervals. Rhythms are said to be produced by variables which oscillate; therefore, the term *oscillation* is often used as a synonym for rhythm. Terms that help describe rhythms are: *peak*, which refers to the maximum value of the oscillating variable; *trough*, which refers to the minimum value; and *cycle*, which is defined as the shortest part of a rhythm that repeats itself indefinitely. A cycle can be measured from any convenient point in one cycle to the corresponding point in the next, i.e., from peak to peak, from trough to trough or between two occurrences of some other easily identifiable point. The *phase* of a rhythm refers to a particular part of a cycle such as the peak or the trough.

Other terms often used by rhythm researchers are period, amplitude and frequency. The *period* of a rhythm is the time occupied by one cycle. The *amplitude* is defined in different ways by different scholars, but is related to the distance from trough to peak. The *frequency* of a rhythm refers to the number of cycles per unit of time. Rhythms with a frequency of approximately once in 24 hours are called circadian rhythms. Ultradian rhythms are rhythms with a period shorter than 24 hours and a frequency of more than once a day. Infradian rhythms are those that have a period longer than 24 hours.

Some rhythms are thought to be dependent upon an external periodicity such as an environmental pattern or cue. These rhythms are described as *exogenous*. In contrast, rhythms are referred to as *endogenous* when the oscillation is considered to originate within the living system. Environmental rhythms thought to influence the rhythms of living systems are called *zeitgebers* (German for time-giver or period-setter). When a zeitgeber is suspended, an endogenous rhythm continues but may show a change in frequency. Such rhythms are referred to as *free-running* (Aschoff 1965, Conroy and Mills 1970, Sollberger 1965).

Rhythms can be divided into two main types, linear and nonlinear. Linear rhythms are best represented by mechanical models such as a pendulum. Nonlinear rhythms are more difficult to represent with mechanical models, although both the siphon and the flexible spring have been used to visually represent characteristics of two distinct types of nonlinear oscillations (Mercer 1965).

The first type of nonlinear rhythm, the relaxation oscillation, has been visually represented by the siphon (Mercer 1965). Relaxation oscillations, like the siphon, build up at differing rates to some critical level and then are discharged. Examples of this kind of rhythm in living systems may be some of the basic physiological and psychological rhythms of hunger, sleep, or anxiety.

The second type of nonlinear rhythm, the limit-cycle oscillation, has been visually represented by the flexible, or nonlinear, spring (Mercer 1965). The child's Slinky® toy is an example of the nonlinear or flexible spring. Rogers (1970) suggested this visual model as an illustration in her early work on the rhythmic nature of living systems. Human rhythms that may be well represented by the limit-cycle model of rhythmic behavior include aspects of consciousness, such as wakefulness or temporality.

The behavior of nonlinear and linear rhythms differs in important respects. For instance, nonlinear oscillations tend to synchronize or couple with each other or with a zeitgeber. There are also differences in the nature of relationships between input and output. With linear rhythms causal relationships between input and output and specific predictions are possible. With nonlinear rhythms outcomes are diverse and can be better discussed in terms of probabilities than in terms of specific predictions (Mercer 1965, Zukav 1979).

The question of the origin of rhythmic phenomena in living systems has stimulated much discussion in the rhythm literature. Are the observed behavioral rhythms generated by living systems and then synchronized with environmental periodicities, or do environmental rhythms stimulate periodicities in living systems? A second question emerges frequently in the debate over the origin of living system rhythms: Is there a "master clock" either within the organism or within the environment that is responsible for the synchronization of rhythms? Although the debate continues, the more recent work of biological researchers suggests that human beings are characterized by a number of interacting, quasi-autonomous, nonlinear rhythms rather than by a central pace-setter or "master clock" (Pavlidis 1978, Vanden Driesche 1973, Winfree 1975).

THE RHYTHM PERSPECTIVE
AND ILLNESS   In discussing health and illness, rhythm theorists have sometimes described illness as the desynchronization of biological rhythms. This desynchronization is postulated to result from the characteristics of endogenous nonlinear oscillations, especially their tendency to free-run with the loss of environmental cues and/or their tendency to couple with other environmental rhythms or with each other.

Within the field of biological psychiatry, attempts have been made to elucidate the relationship between desynchronized circadian rhythms and mental illness. It is still not known whether there are mental illnesses specifically related to changes in circadian organization. The hypothesis of desynchronized circadian rhythms, however, underlies much psychiatric theorizing.

Desynchronization theory has been considered a useful working hypothesis by clinical researchers focusing on affective illness. The attraction of the theory is related to its ability to explain a number of clinical observations. For instance, a desynchronization of biological rhythms would explain the gradual development and symmetric course of many affective disturbances. The diurnal variation in symptoms often reported in affective disturbances can also be associated with desynchronization of circadian rhythms, since the ratio between two variables out of their usual phase relationship will change during the day. The increased incidence of depressions in spring and autumn can also be related to desynchronized circadian rhythms if one considers the possibility of certain rhythms beginning to free-run in response to the respective increase and decrease in the days length (Mellerup and Rafaelsen 1979).

The heuristic value of the desynchronization theory is further increased by its ability to explain the clinical effectiveness of various treatment approaches used for affective illnesses. The effect of phase advancing the sleep-wake cycle (Wehr et al. 1979) and of sleep deprivation (Milstein et al. 1979, Rudolf and Tölle 1978) on the depressive symptoms can be explained by postulating a resynchronization process between biological variables closely linked to the sleep-wake cycle and other less closely linked variables. When the sleep-wake cycle is shifted, those variables closely linked to the cycle are thought to shift also. This results in the establishment of a new phase relationship with the less closely linked variables, e.g., those that continue in their established rhythm. Treatment of depression using mood elevators is also explained by the drugs' effect on the sleep-wake cycle. Lithium's observed ability to change the lengths of various circadian periods is thought to counteract a desynchronization of biological rhythms and thereby prevent affective episodes (Mellerup and Rafaelsen 1979).

Richter (1965) has taken a different view of the way rhythms interact. He also describes the human body as possessing or being a multiple, self-sustained set of interacting oscillators; however, he conceptualizes desynchronization as necessary to the maintenance of smooth performance. He suggests that each part of the organism may have a similar intrinsic rhythm and that smooth functioning of the organism depends on random phase relationships. Richter's "shock phase hypothesis" sets forth the idea that psychosis arises from the synchronization of rhythms following an insult. Such an insult is hypothesized to synchronize the similar intrinsic rhythms of each part, resulting in the uniform pathological oscillation of the whole organism.

Stroebel (1967) also has explored the relationship between circadian rhythms and mental illness. He has reported that deconditioning is much more efficient if performed at the time of day at which conditioning has occurred. Stroebel (1969) also found that severe stress could lead to desynchronization of rhythms. In his animal studies, primates who were stressed responded in one of two ways: (1) with desynchronized circadian rhythms of temperature accompanied by physical disorders; or (2) by developing new 48-hour temperature rhythms. The group with desynchronized temperature rhythms with accompanying physical disorders were reported to return to normal when stressors were removed or when tranquilizing agents were given; those with 48-hour rhythms were more likely to persist in their new pattern.

The unreformulated rhythm perspective has implications for the treatment of illness using the traditional medical model. In the traditional medical model, illness is viewed as a biological system disturbance residing within the person; treatment consists of altering internal processes. For example, a nurse working with depressed clients utilizing the unreformulated rhythm perspective within a medical model would likely focus on therapy designed to alter the phase relationships of internal rhythms and thereby lift the depression. Thus, the sleep pattern of the person might be manipulated and/or the nurse might seek to have mood elevators prescribed by a physician. The focus of the nurse-client relationship would most likely be the environmental stressors thought to have disrupted internal rhythms.

THE RHYTHM PERSPECTIVE
AND HEALTH   The rhythms of healthy human functioning also have received attention. Kleitman (1963) proposed a basic rest activity cycle (BRAC) continuing throughout the 24-hour day with sleep and wakefulness superimposed upon it. His choice of terms, i.e., "rest" and "activity" have been questioned (Kripke 1974). Nevertheless, Kleitman's suggestion of a generalized rhythm modulating behavioral functions throughout the 24-hour period has inspired a number of studies.

One of the first researchers to explore the idea of an ultradian rhythm persisting throughout the 24-hour day was Globus. He explored rhythms of gross motor activity, electroencephalography rhythms, and the rhythmic responses to the Rorschach test. Ultradian rhythms of daydreaming have also been explored (Kripke and Sonnenshein 1978), as well as studies of the timing of eating, drinking, and smoking. Cycles in oral behavior were found by Friedman and Fisher (1967) and Oswald et al. (1970). Friedman also explored orality cycles in obese persons (1972). In most of these studies, rhythms with cycles of 90-120 minutes have been reported.

Recently, it has been hypothesized that ultradian rhythms involve an alteration in the relative efficiency of the two cerebral hemispheres. In one of the more recent studies (Klein and Armitage 1979), performance on verbal and spatial matching tasks was assessed every 15 minutes for eight hours. Significant 90- to 100-minute rhythms were observed for each task. These oscillations were reported to be 180 degrees out of phase with each other, i.e., verbal performance peaked when spatial matching had its lowest value and vice versa. The data were interpreted to support the hypothesis that, in humans, the basic rest activity cycle involves alternating activation of processing systems residing in the two cerebral hemispheres.

Systematic work on emotional rhythms in healthy populations also has been reported. Hersey (1931) studied factory workers and found both daily and monthly rhythms in emotional tone. In more recent studies daily mood variation has been studied in other populations. In general, in adults positive moods are reported to increase and negative moods decrease at midday and late afternoon compared to morning (Taub and Berger 1974). The opposite trend has been reported with adolescents (Barton 1974).

Some of the most interesting work on the rhythms of healthy human functioning has been reported by Halberg and his associates (Halberg et al. 1973). They have attempted to develop inexpensive practical methods for evaluating fluctuations in biological and psychological variables. Halberg calls his approach "autorhythmometry." It involves the training of subjects in self-assessment of daily changes in mood and time perception as well as measuring and assessing one's own blood pressure, pulse, temperature, and grip strength. Halberg suggests his approach will find application in the area of preventive medicine since early detection of alterations in one or more rhythms could be used to alert the individual to the need for professional evaluation.

The unreformulated rhythm perspective has implications for the prevention of illness using the ecological model. The ecological or public health model (Phillips 1977) considers health and illness as the result of agent-host-environment interaction. Prevention and early detection of illness are primary aims in this model. For example, nurses utilizing the unreformulated rhythm perspective within an ecological model might deal with depression as a health problem by identifying high-risk individuals and teaching them to monitor their own rhythms. In addition, clients at risk might be helped to develop new interactional patterns to alter some aspect of themselves or their environments, thus reducing stress and the accompanying desynchronization of rhythms.

The research and practice just described illustrate the variety of approaches being taken to explore rhythmicity and its relationship to health and illness. Although these approaches have implications for nursing, they do not reflect the unique perspective of nursing. The unique contribution of nursing emerges when borrowed frameworks are reformulated. Therefore, the rhythm perspective developing within related disciplines will be reformulated within the nursing models of Rogers and Newman.

REFORMULATION WITHIN ROGERS' CONCEPTUAL MODEL

Within Rogers' conceptual model, man and environment are defined as four-dimensional, negentropic energy fields identified by pattern and organization. The model emphasizes the reasoning and feeling nature of human beings and postulates that human beings have the capacity to participate knowingly and probabilistically in the process of change. Each human being is unique. Each person's environment also is unique since it encompasses all that is outside any given person (Rogers 1970).

Three principles, resonancy, helicy, and complementarity, are central to Rogers' (1980) conceptualization. Only the principles of resonancy and helicy are emphasized here; complementarity is considered later. The principle of resonancy describes how change occurs. It denotes a rhythmic flow of waveforms that order and reorder the human and environmental fields. According to Rogers, rhythmicity is a concomitant of life and its environment. The life process is described as proceeding rhythmically along a spiraling axis, with each new curve of the spiral revealing cyclical continuity rather than repetition. Rhythmic phenomena are viewed as expressions of the complementary relationship between man and environment with the rhythms of life being inextricably woven into the rhythms of the universe (Rogers 1970, 1980).

The principle of helicy describes the nature and direction of change, which is toward increasing complexity and diversity of human field pattern and organization and toward waveforms of increasing frequency. Any rhythmic process can be considered as increasing in complexity if it incorporates increasingly more units in its pattern and organization. If the units are the same as those initially present, the increase in complexity can be described as a quantitative change. If the units are different from those initially present, the increase in complexity involves a change in form, that is, a qualitative change (Lerner 1976). While increasing complexity manifests itself within a given human or environmental field, diversity manifests itself across fields. When examining some characteristic of a number of human or environmental fields, one can say there is increasing diversity when fields manifest greater variety, that is, the kinds of waveform patterning and organization increase.

Rogers describes life's rhythms as integral to and inseparable from environmental rhythms. Deviations in the rhythmic relationship between man and environment are postulated to manifest themselves in disruption and reorganization of the human field and the environmental field directed toward the evolution of new rhythmical relationships. These new rhythmical relationships are described as innovative, probabilistic, and embedded in the man-environment interaction. They are characterized by increasing complexity and diversity of waveform pattern and organization.

In Rogers' model, increasing complexity and diversity are not synonomous with health as health is commonly understood. According to Rogers, health and illness typically have been thought of dichotomously and are value-laden terms. Rogers, however, describes health and illness as part of the same continuum rather than as dichotomous conditions. All conditions, whatever their nature or label of health or illness, are probabilistic expressions of the person-environment interaction.

The major correlate of mental health and illness as defined within the rhythm framework and Rogers' model is rhythmic phenomena. The congruencies and incongruencies between Rogers' model and the rhythm perspective will be discussed in relationship to this correlate. Considering congruencies first, both frameworks postulate the rhythmic nature of man and environment and identify change as occurring through waveform repatterning. Both frameworks conceptualize man as an open system characterized by nonlinear waveforms. In addition, both postulate probabilistic outcomes in development.

There are also incongruencies between the two frameworks requiring a reformulation of the rhythm perspective if it is to be congruent with Rogers' conceptual model. The major incongruency is the failure within the rhythm perspective to conceptualize the environment as an open system. The environment is frequently conceptualized as rhythmic by scholars in the field, but the consequence of this rhythmicity (that the environment cannot be a closed system) has not been emphasized. Failure to emphasize the environment as an open system results in little attention to the mutuality involved in man-environment interaction. Rogers (1980) does emphasize this mutuality, identifying a third principle, complementarity, which is subsumed under helicy but extracted from it to emphasize the acausal nature of person-environment evolution.

The de-emphasis of the environment as an open system within the rhythm perspective is obvious in the exploration of mental health and mental illness. In this area much more emphasis has been placed on the within-person or psychological and physiological correlates of behavior than on the environmental correlates. Even when the environmental correlates have been addressed, there has been a major emphasis on physical rhythms of the environment rather than the environment as defined by Rogers, which includes cultural, social, and interpersonal rhythms encompassing values, ideas, and emotions.

A second incongruency is the lack of any postulate within the rhythmic perspective encompassing the direction of change in waveform repatterning. Rogers' principle of helicy identifies the direction of change, but within the rhythm framework no similar principle has been developed and, therefore, without reformulation no predictions can be made about the developmental outcomes of waveform repatterning beyond the statement that they are probabilistic.

A third incongruency between the rhythm perspective and Rogers' model is Rogers' focus on the rhythmic activity of indices of the whole person, i.e., human field rhythms or rhythms of synergistic functioning. Thus far, the majority of rhythm researchers outside of nursing have focused upon particulate rhythms, i.e., physiological, biological, or psychological rhythms.

In summary, the reformulation of the rhythm perspective that is necessary to make it congruent with Rogers' conceptual model requires three changes: (1) the environmental field must be defined as an open system that is different for each person; (2) a postulate stating the direction of change in waveform repatterning as being toward increasing complexity and diversity must be included; and (3) a shift in emphasis away from particulate and toward holistic rhythms is required.

REFORMULATION WITHIN NEWMAN'S
CONCEPTUAL MODEL
Newman's (1979) conceptual model of health is based on an open systems model of person-environment interaction. Life is described as being composed of the energy of matter and motion each of which can be transformed into the other. Drawing from the recent theory building advances of particle physicists, Newman notes that particles have no meaning as isolated entities, but only as interrelated changing events. From this she concludes that, "the world . . . must be viewed as a complicated network of interrelated changing events, as dynamic patterns of activity, with space aspects and time aspects" (1979, p. 60).

In Newman's model, an understanding of health is built upon the interrelationship among four concepts: movement, time, space, and consciousness. Movement is described in three ways: first, as an essential property of matter; second, as a means by which space and time become a reality; and third, as a reflection of consciousness. In explicating these ideas, Newman discusses an "action-rest cycle," which is manifest in many ways including the firing of neurons, the contraction of muscle tissue and the patterns of language and body movement. Drawing again from the "new physics" Newman notes that change between two states of rest, i.e., rest-action-rest, is a requirement for manifest reality. Thus, in Newman's model, rhythmicity is necessary for the person's sense of time and space; this subjective sense of time and space represents consciousness. Newman conceptualizes health as the expansion of consciousness. Therefore, rhythmicity, which undergirds the person's consciousness, is integrally related to health in Newman's model. Health as conceptualized by Newman encompasses conditions which have been described as pathological. Building on Rogers' assumption that pattern and organization identify human energy fields, Newman describes the pattern of the individual as primary. This pattern exists prior to structural or functional changes described as pathology. Therefore, removal of the pathology in itself will not change the pattern of the person. According to Newman, "if becoming ill is the only way an individual's pattern can manifest itself, then that is health for that person" (1979, p. 58).

Congruencies between Newman's conceptual model of health and the rhythm perspective can be identified. For instance, both frameworks conceptualize the person as an open system characterized by rhythmicity and both models view rhythmicity as a correlate of health and illness. There are also incongruencies between the two frameworks. The most noticeable difference is Newman's focus on macrorhythms, i.e., larger or whole-person rhythms of movement, as opposed to rhythm researchers' focus on microrhythms, i.e., psychological, biological, or physiological rhythms. An additional difference is Newman's clear emphasis on the relationship between rhythmicity and temporal and spatial experience. Although empirical evidence of altered temporal and spatial experience during major mental disturbance abounds, rhythm researchers in the mental health disciplines have not addressed the theoretical significance of these findings.

Since Newman's conceptualization of health was derived within an open systems model, the reformulation of rhythm theory necessary to achieve congruency with Rogers' conceptual model is consistent with Newman's formulation. An additional modification of the rhythm perspective suggested by Newman's work is a postulate regarding rhythms as intrinsically related to the temporal and spatial aspects of consciousness.

RELATIONSHIP OF THE RHYTHM PERSPECTIVE
TO THE MODELS OF KING,
OREM, AND ROY   Rhythmic activity is not an explicit aspect of the nursing models of King (1971), Orem (1980), or Roy (1976). Although this observation precludes reformulation of the rhythm perspective within the models of King, Orem, or Roy, it is possible to identify points of articulation between the rhythm perspective and these nursing models. For instance, King's (1971) discussion of the nursing process of action, reaction, interaction, and transaction suggests rhythmicity. Subsequent work on nurse-patient interaction has explored the rhythmic nature of verbal and nonverbal behavior within the nurse-client relationship. For instance, Daubenmire et al. (1978) have reported work on the development of a methodological framework for exploring the rhythmic patterns of verbal and nonverbal behavior. Basic to this methodological framework, which is called "synchronology," are the concepts of convergence and divergence. "Convergence denotes a process of increasing behavior similarity. Divergence denotes decreasing similarity of behavior" (p. 308). Communication rhythms are described as converging, diverging, or remaining stationary as the nurse and client interact over time.

Both King (1971) and Daubenmire et al. (1978) describe the nursing process in a manner consistent with an understanding of communication rhythms as nonlinear oscillations. Thus, the methodological framework of Daubenmire et al. can be conceptualized as a methodology for the study of coupling or synchronizing behavior among nonlinear waveforms.

Orem's model (1980) focuses on the concept of self care in its various forms. A linkage between the concept of rhythmicity and Orem's model emerges around the influence of various rhythms, including physiological and psychological rhythms, on self-care requirements and self care agency. Since rhythm researchers have begun to explicate the relationships between various particulate rhythms and human performance (Colquhoun 1971), the rhythm perspective can contribute a great deal to the nurse's understanding of fluctuation in self care requirements and self-care agency. For utilization within Orem's model, the rhythm perspective does not require reformulation. Many of the contributions of the unreformulated framework are discussed in the next section describing implications for practice.

Points of articulation between Roy's model (1976) and rhythm theory are difficult to identify since the classical concept of adaptation is antithetical to the concept of rhythmicity. Using the rhythm perspective within the Roy model would require a reconceptualization of adaptation, moving away from the sense of human beings maintaining relative balance by adjusting to environmental impingements.

IMPLICATIONS OF THE RHYTHM PERSPECTIVE
FOR PROFESSIONAL PRACTICE   In the past decade, a number of authors have discussed ways in which an understanding of rhythmic phenomena relates to the practice of nursing. One of the earliest researchers in nursing to publish regarding rhythmic phenomena was Felton (1970, 1973, 1975, Felton and Ward 1977).

In writing about the relationship between an understanding of rhythmicity and patient care, Felton (1970) recommended a "spectral" or "range" view when considering physiological change in parameters such as blood pressure and body temperature. She defined this view as one that "looks for a uniformity of function along a continuum of relationships with an upper and a lower limit between the occurrence of a peak (high) or a trough (low) in the daily curve" (p. 57). As Felton pointed out, a particular blood pressure or temperature reading might be within expected limits during one phase of the circadian rhythm, but above or below the expected limits during another phase. Her research also suggested that the particular timing of peaks and troughs was meaningful only if the person's mode of life was also defined since rhythmic behavior often changed with a change in the mode of life (Felton 1970).

Felton has consistently addressed the relationship among social, psychological, and physiological rhythms in her research and publications and has underscored the importance of regarding "time" as a dimension of experience for both the provider and recipient of nursing care. With regard to practicing nurses, Felton has frequently discussed the relationship between understanding human rhythmicity and nursing practice. Felton (1975) suggests that many performance factors including job satisfaction, medication errors, and errors in problem solving, can be related to the nurse's circadian cycle.

A large collection of articles on biological rhythms was published in 1976 in *Nursing Clinics of North America* (Tom and Lanuza 1976). Each of the authors publishing in this symposium addressed implications of the rhythm perspective for nursing practice. For instance, Lanuza (1976) noted that the nurse's awareness of rhythms should play an important role in planning with patients the best time for scheduling patient-teaching sessions, rehabilitation exercises, activities of daily living, and various treatment procedures, as well as rest periods. In the area of patient-teaching, she specifically identified the importance of instructing patients regarding the effects of shift-work and jet lag on sleep patterns, appetite, gastrointestinal functioning, and susceptibility to medication.

Tom (1976) emphasized nursing assessment of biological rhythms identifying a number of questions to be asked regarding patients' physical, psychological, and social rhythms. She divided these questions into two categories. The first category consists of those questions that generate objective data; the second category consists of questions generating subjective data. Objective data consist of information regarding the rhythmic qualities of vital signs, intake and output, blood values, changes in mood, life stress, usual activity schedule, and activity schedule imposed by illness. Tom notes that most of what she categorized as objective data were data that nurses already collect on their patients. It is the interpretation of these data that she suggests requires a new focus. Subjective data consist of information obtained by the patient's self report and are sought to give clues to the patient's individual circadian patterns. The questions asked center around the patient's view of himself as a "day" or "night" person and the ease with which he can shift these rhythms.

Tom has identified three areas where rhythm data can be used. A major area is referred to as "environmental control" and consists of planning nursing care procedures, meals and rest-activity schedules considering the patient's circadian rhythms rather than hospital staff's convenience. A second area is that of scheduling medication administration for optimal times. These optimal times have been documented to correlate with circadian patterns of temperature, serum cortisol levels, and activity (Smolensky and Reinberg 1976). The third area is to gain insight into the nurse's own rhythms and their influence on her work performance and nurse-patient interactions.

Bassler (1976) considered nursing implications of the rhythm perspective for the nursing care of children. She views the nurse as a "primary mediator between the patient and his environment." As such, the nurse caring for an infant or young child can promote rhythm development. Bassler outlined suggestions for both assessment and intervention. These include: (1) the careful monitoring of physiological functions with early detection of desynchronization of these rhythms; (2) the monitoring of expressions of temporal experience as potential clues to behavioral disturbances; (3) the determination of sleep-wakefulness patterns demonstrated by the child both at home and in the health care setting for the purposes of noting changes in patterns caused by a change of environments and to create a care environment supportive of previously established patterns; (4) the assessment of social structure in the family unit for the purpose of preserving the child's established routine during hospitalization, and thus, possibly preventing the disruption of developing rhythms; and (5) the assessment of the effect of environments, such as intensive care nurseries, on rhythm development.

Hall (1976) has written about the nursing implications of the rhythm perspective in the area of geriatric nursing. Working specifically in the area of rehabilitation of the chronically ill aged, she found that the temperature rhythm was helpful in planning the time for rehabilitation activities in the motor-kinetic ability area although language and cognitive learning patterns did not run parallel. She also noted that rhythmicity information seemed useful in decreasing tension and frustration. Thus, synchronizing the rehabilitation activities appeared to lead to more steady, although not necessarily more rapid, progress.

Since the articles on biological rhythms published in 1976 in *Nursing Clinics of North America*, a few nurses have published research on rhythmic phenomena and have discussed ways in which an understanding of rhythmicity relates to nursing practice. For instance, Leddy (1977) reported a study in which she explored the relationship between sleep and phase shifting of biologic variables. Leddy assumed that "normal" body rhythms were associated with the "healthy state" and that nursing is concerned with the maintenance and restoration of health. Thus Leddy recommended that nurses aid in restoration of healthy relationships among biological variables and sleep-wake patterns by individualizing hospital routines. Her own research has explored the relationships among sleep and phase shifting of blood pressure and temperature rhythms.

Hoskins (1979) has studied family relationships focusing on rhythms. She emphasizes the importance of knowledge of the temporal aspects of family relationships when assessing family process and has stated that effective intervention with troubled families will require a broad theoretical base of knowledge, including a rhythm perspective. Her research has explored the relationship among differing energy level and body temperature rhythms of family members and interpersonal conflict in family relationships.

IMPLICATIONS OF THE REFORMULATED FRAMEWORK FOR PRACTICE AND RESEARCH   Many of the implications for nursing practice described above have emphasized the usefulness of the rhythm perspective without explicit reformulation. Since the professional practice of any discipline draws from a broad base of knowledge, this is consistent with sound clinical practice (Donaldson and Crowley 1978). However, the importance of reformulating existing frameworks to facilitate the development of the discipline of nursing has been described in the introduction. Therefore the implications of the reformulated framework for practice and research are discussed.

Utilization of the reformulated rhythm perspective within Rogers' model can influence nursing practice in a number of ways. The data base needed for professional practice would include an assessment of human field rhythmicities in addition to the usual assessment of biological, psychological, and social rhythms. Rogers has suggested that individual rhythm profiles might become standard diagnostic data. The assessments using this reformulated framework would be based upon an understanding of the probabilistic nature rather than a causal nature of developmental outcomes. The interventions using this reformulation would be based on an understanding of the postulated nature and direction of waveform repatterning. They would include the conscious manipulation of environmental rhythmicities including cultural, social, interpersonal, and physical patterns of the environment for the purpose of intervening in human field repatterning.

As an example, a nurse utilizing the reformulated rhythm perspective with depressed persons would view the behavioral pattern as an expression of the person-environment interaction. The rhythmic patterns of communication, mood, wakefulness, temporality, and movement would be explored along with their unique interplay within the person's life space. As an understanding of the relationships among these human field rhythms emerged, the person could knowingly participate in the alteration of selected rhythmic patterns. For instance, the person might choose to alter his patterns of physical exercise, sleep, meditation, or communication and note corresponding shifts in patterns of mood. Since the practice of any professional discipline draws from the knowledge base of related fields (Donaldson and Crowley 1978), intervention would not be limited to the focus on human field rhythms, and might also include the conscious altering of social, psychological, or biological rhythms.

A nurse utilizing the rhythm perspective as reformulated within Newman's model would view the person's behavior as an expression of his pattern and organization. In the case of depression, for instance, the behavioral patterns might be seen as health for the person in the sense that they represent the only way the individual's pattern can manifest itself at the moment. One focus of data collection and assessment would be the temporal and spatial aspects of the person's conscious experience which, in the case of depression, is marked by altered mood. Another focus would be the relationship of the person's patterns of movement to his conscious experience of altered mood. With depressed persons, patterns of movement might be marked by either lethargy or agitation. Interventions which are understood to alter one's rhythmic sense of space, time, or movement might be incorporated by nurses utilizing the rhythm perspective as reformulated within Newman's model.

A specific clinical example is a middle-aged woman who has come to a community mental health center seeking assistance with multiple difficulties. These difficulties include feelings of inadequacy and time pressure regarding her performance in a new job outside the home, feelings of helplessness and anger in relation to a teen-aged son's rebellious behavior, elevated blood pressure, and obesity. The nurse, using a rhythm perspective reformulated within Rogers' and Newman's models, might begin by establishing a data base including a rhythm profile. The rhythm profile would include patterns of most concern to the client. For instance, keeping a log of daily variations in mood, sense of time passing, usual activity, and communication patterns might be recommended. For this client, the recording of variations in feelings of hunger, thoughts about food, and blood pressure might also be recommended. The interaction among these rhythms would be studied and the client could begin to alter one or more of the rhythmic patterns and note the developing outcomes in relation to other rhythms. She might find a change in her sleep-wake cycle or physical exercise cycle is related to mood or that changes in her communication patterns are related to an increase in energy, lower blood pressure readings, or fewer thoughts of food. Other possibilities include a connection between increased physical activity and a decreased sense of time passing too quickly, or changes in her communication patterns with her son and an improved mood. Whatever the nature of the interacting patterns for this client, the emphasis would be on her participating consciously in her own repatterning.

As this example demonstrates well, the needed knowledge base for this nursing approach is in its infancy. What is needed at the present time is a great deal more clinical nursing research to establish likely relationships among human field and particulate rhythms as well as the probabilities of various outcomes when attempts at changing rhythmic patterns are made.

Research and theory development in psychiatric mental health nursing will benefit from the testing of reformulations of existing frameworks within nursing's conceptual models. A number of areas of research in psychiatric mental health nursing are suggested by the reformulation of the rhythm perspective within Rogers and Newman's models. Work on the rhythm perspective in nursing has begun: e.g., Felton's (1970, 1973, 1976) and Hoskins' (1979) research cited earlier; Fitzpatrick's (1978, 1980), Newman's (1976, 1979), and Tomkins' (1980) research on temporal experience and motion; and Neal's (1968, 1976) research on motion and infant development. Thus far, few nurse researchers have related their studies of rhythmic phenomena to psychiatric populations. One exception is Fitzpatrick, who has focused on temporal experience during crisis (Fitzpatrick 1980, Fitzpatrick et al. 1980).

SUMMARY   The goal of this chapter has been to draw attention to the potential usefulness of the rhythm perspective for psychiatric mental health nursing. The position has been taken that the unreformulated rhythm perspective has many implications for the psychiatric mental health disciplines. In addition, when the rhythm perspective is reformulated within nursing's conceptual system, it can guide both practice and research in nursing. The basic tenets of the rhythm perspective necessitate an open systems model for reformulation. Therefore, Rogers' and Newman's conceptual models are utilized for the actual reformulation, although other models are also discussed.

References

Aschoff J: Circadian Clocks, Amsterdam. North-Holland, 1965

Auger JA: Physiological issues in mental health nursing. *In* Leininger M (Ed.): Contemporary Issues in Mental Health Nursing, Boston, Little, Brown & Company, 1973

Barton K, Cattell RB: Changes in psychological state measures and time of day. Psycholog Rep, 35:219–222, 1974

Bassler SF: The origins and development of biological rhythms. Nursing Clinics of North America, 11:575–582, 1976

Colquhoun WP (Ed.): Biological Rhythms and Human Performance, New York, Academic Press, 1971

Conroy RT, Mills JN: Human Circadian Rhythms, London. J. & A. Churchill, 1970

Daubenmire MJ, Searles SS, Ashton CA: A methodological framework to study nurse-patient communication. Nurs Res, 27:303–310, 1978

Donaldson S, Crowley. The discipline of nursing. Nurs Outlook, 26:113–120, 1978

Fagin CM: Psychotherapeutic nursing. Am J Nurs, 67:298–304, 1967

Fawcett J: A framework for analysis and evaluation of conceptual models of nursing. Nurse Educator, November-December:10–14, 1980

Fawcett J: The what of theory development. *In* Theory Development: What, Why, and How, New York, National League for Nursing, 1978

Felton G: Effect of time cycle change on blood pressure and temperature in young women. Nurs Res, 19:48–58, 1970

Felton G: Rhythmic correlates of shift work. *In* Batey MV (Ed.): Communicating Nursing Research (Vol. 6), Boulder, Western Interstate Commission for Higher Education, 1973

Felton G: Body rhythm effects on rotating work shifts. Nurs Dig, 4:29–32, 1976

Felton G, Ward J: Regression models in the study of circadian rhythms in nursing research. Int J Nurs Stud, 14:151–161, 1977

Fitzpatrick JJ: Patients' perceptions of time: current research. Int Nurs Rev, 27:148–153, 1980

Fitzpatrick JJ, Donovan MJ: Temporal experience and motor behavior among the aging. Res Nurs Health, 1:60–68, 1978

Fitzpatrick JJ, Donovan MJ, Johnston RL: Experience of time during crisis of cancer. J Cancer Nurs, 3:191–194, 1980

Fitzpatrick JJ, Johnston RL, Donovan MJ: Hospitalization as a crisis: Relation to temporal experience (Abst.). In WICHE Proceedings. Communicating Nursing Research Directions for the 1980's, Vol XIII, 1980

Flaskerud JH, Holleran EJ: Areas of agreement in nursing theory development. Adv Nurs Sci, 3:1–7, 1980

Friedman S: On the presence of a variant form of instinctual regression: oral drive cycles in obesity-bulimia. Psychoanalyt Quart, 41:364–383, 1972

Friedman S, Fisher C: On the presence of a rhythmic, diurnal, oral, instinctual drive cycle in man: a preliminary report. J. Am Psychoanal. Assoc., 225:959–960, 1967

Globus GG: Observations on sub-circadian rhythms. Psychophysiology, 4:366, 1968

Globus GG: Rapid eye movement cycle in real time. Arch Gen Psychiatry, 15:654–659, 1966

Globus GG, Drury RI, Phoebus EC, Boyd R: Ultradian rhythms in human performance. Percept Mot Skills, 33:1171–1174, 1971

Halberg F, Johnson EA, Nelson W, Sothern R: Autorythmometry: procedures for physiologic self-assessment and their analysis. Physiol Teacher, 1:1–4, 1973

Hall LH: Circadian rhythms: implications for geriatric rehabilitation. Nurs Clin North Am, 11:631–638, 1976

Hersey RB: Workers Emotions in Shop and Home, Philadelphia, University of Pennsylvania Press, 1932

Hoskins CN: Level of activation, body temperature, and interpersonal conflict in family relationships. Nurs Res, 28:154–160, 1979

Johnson D: Development of theory: a requisite for nursing as a primary health profession. Nurs Res, 23:372–376, 1974

King IM: Toward a Theory for Nursing, New York, John Wiley & Sons, Inc., 1971

Klein R, Armitage R: Rhythms in human performance: 1½-hour oscillations in cognitive style. Science, 204:1326–1328, 1979

Kleitman N: Sleep and Wakefulness (rev. ed.), Chicago, University of Chicago Press, 1963

Kripke D: Ultradian rhythms in sleep and wakefulness. In Weitsman E (Ed.), Advances in Sleep Research (Vol. 1). New York, Spectrum Publications, 1974

Kripke DF, Sonnenshein D, in K. Pope and J. Singer (Eds.): The Stream of Consciousness, New York, Plenum, 1978

Lanuza DM: Circadian rhythms of mental efficiency and performance. Nurs Clin North Am, 11:583–594, 1976

Leddy S: Sleep and phase shifting of biological rhythms. Int J Nurs Stud, 14:137–150, 1977

Lego S: Nurse psychotherapists: How are we different? Perspect Psychiatr Care, 11:144–147, 1973

Leininger MM (Ed.): Contemporary Issues in Mental Health Nursing. Boston, Little, Brown & Company, 1973

Lerner R: Concepts and Theories of Human Development, Reading, Massachusetts, Addison-Wesley, 1976

Mellerup ET, Rafaelsen OJ: Circadian rhythms in manic-melancholic disorders. Current Developments in Psychopharmacology, 51–66, 1979

Mellow J: Nursing therapy. Am J Nurs, 68:2365–2369, 1968

Mercer M: In Aschoff J: Circadian Clocks, Amsterdam, North-Holland, 1965

Milstein V, Small JG, Sharpley P, Golay S: All night sleep deprivation in psychiatric patients: relation to mood, EEG, and psychiatric diagnosis. Clin Electroencephalogr, 10:25–30, 1979

Muller TG: Nature and Direction of Psychiatric Nursing, Philadelphia, Lippincott, 1950

Neal MV: Vestibular stimulation and developmental behavior of the small premature infant. Nurs Res Rep. New York, American Nurses Foundation, March, 1968

Neal MV (Ed.): The Conceptual Basis for Maternal Child Health Nursing Practice, Baltimore, University of Maryland, 1976

Newman MA: Movement tempo and the experience of time. Nurs Res, 25:273–279, 1976

Newman MA: Theory Development in Nursing, Philadelphia, F. A. Davis, 1979

Orem DE: Nursing: Concepts of practice (2nd ed.), New York, McGraw-Hill Book Company, 1980

Osborne OH: Anthropological issues in mental health nursing. In Leininger M (Ed.): Contemporary Issues in Mental Health Nursing, Boston, Little, Brown & Company, 1973

Oswald I, Merrington J, Lewis H: Cyclical "on demand" oral intake by adults. Nature, 225:959–960, 1970

Paterson JG, Zderad LT: Humanistic Nursing, New York, John Wiley & Sons, 1976

Pavladis T: What do mathematical models tell us about circadian clocks? Bull Math Biol, 40:625–635, 1978

Peplau HE: Interpersonal Relations in Nursing, New York, G. P. Putnam's Sons, 1952

Phillips JR: Nursing systems and nursing models. Image, 9:4–7, 1977

Pothier PC: Sensory integration therapy. *In* Kneisl C, Wilson H (Eds.): Current Perspectives in Psychiatric Nursing: Issues and Trends (Vol. 2), St. Louis, The C. V. Mosby Company, 1978

Richter CP: Biological Clocks in Medicine and Psychiatry, Springfield, Ill., Thomas, 1965

Rogers ME: An Introduction to the Theoretical Basis of Nursing, Philadelphia, F. A. Davis, 1970

Rogers M: Nursing: a science of unitary man. *In* Riehl J, Roy C (Eds.): Conceptual Models for Nursing Practice (2nd ed.), New York, Appleton-Century-Crofts, 1980

Roy C: Introduction to Nursing: An Adaptation Model, Englewood Cliffs, New Jersey, Prentice-Hall, Inc., 1976

Rudolf GAE, Tölle R: Sleep deprivation and circadian rhythm in depression. Psychiatr Clin (Basel), 11:198–212, 1978

Sayre J: The new therapies and the search for the "real" self. *In* Kneisl C, Wilson H (Eds.): Current Perspectives in Psychiatric Nursing: Issues and Trends (Vol. 2), St. Louis, The C. V. Mosby Company, 1978

Smolensky MH, Reinberg A: The chronotherapy of corticosteroids: practical application of chronobiological findings to nursing. Nurs Clin North Am, 11:609–620, 1976

Sollberger A: Biological Rhythm Research, Amsterdam, Elsevier Publishing Company, 1965

Stephens GJ: Periodicity in mood, affect, and instinctual behavior. Nurs Clin North Am, 11:595–607, 1976

Stroebel CF: Behavioral aspects of circadian rhythms. *In* Zulim J, Hu HF (Eds.): Comparative Psychopathology, Animal, and Human, New York, Grume & Stratton, pp. 158–172, 1967

Stroebel CF: Biologic rhythm correlates of disturbed behavior in the rhesus monkey. Bibl Primatol, 9:91–105, 1969

Taub MJ, Berger RJ: Performance and mood following variations in the length and timing of sleep. Psychophysiology, 10:559–570, 1973

Tom CK: Nursing assessment of biological rhythms. Nurs Clin North Am, 11:621–630, 1976

Tom CK, Lanuza DM: Symposium of biological rhythms. Nurs Clin North Am, 11:569–573, 1976

Tompkins ES: Effect of restricted mobility and dominance on perceived duration. Nurs Res, 29:333–338, 1980

Ujhely GB: The nurse as psychotherapist: what are the issues. Perspect Psychiatr Care, 11:155–160, 1973

Vanden Driesche T: A population of oscillators: a working hypothesis and its compatibility with experimental evidence. Int J Chronobiol, 1:253–258, 1973

Wehr TA, Wirz-Justice A, Goodwin FK, Duncan W, Gillin JC: Phase advance of the circadian sleep-wake cycle as an anti-depressant. Science, 206:710–713, 1979

Whall A: Congruence between family theory and nursing models. Adv Nurs Sci, 3:59–67, 1980

Winfree AT: Unclocklike behavior of biological clocks. Nature, 253:315–319, 1975

Zukav G: The Dancing Wu Li Masters: An Overview of the New Physics, New York, William Morrow & Company, 1979

AUTHOR INDEX

Orem   2, 4, 6, 7, 12, 13, 16, 30, 32,
   33, 38, 56, 57, 58, 69, 70, 82–84,
   91, 106
Osborne   96
Oswald et al.   101

Parad and Caplan   71
Paterson and Zderad   96
Pavlidis   98
Peplau   1, 2, 38, 43, 47, 53–56, 95
Phillips   101
Pothier   96

Rank   1
Rappoport   20
Richter   99
Rogers   2, 4, 6–10, 16, 30, 33, 34,
   38, 53, 64–66, 69, 70, 81, 86–90,
   96–98, 102–105, 109, 111
Roy   2, 4, 6, 7, 14–16, 30–33, 38,
   61, 62, 69, 81, 82, 84–86, 90, 91,
   106

Sayre   96
Schlotfeldt   16
Sills   2
Smolensky and Reinberg   108

Smoyak   72
Sollberger   97
Stephens   96
Stroebel   100
Sullivan   39, 40–45, 47, 58, 62

Taplin   27–29, 31
Taub and Berger   101
Tom   107
Tom and Lanuza   107
Tomkins   111
Tudor   2
Tyhurst   20

Ujhely   95

vanden Driesche   98
von Bertalanffy   5

Watzlawick et al.   12, 50, 64
Weakland   50
Wehr et al.   99
Wells et al.   91
Whall   3, 4, 7, 69, 95
Winfree   98

Zukav   98

SUBJECT INDEX